Red Socks Don't Work

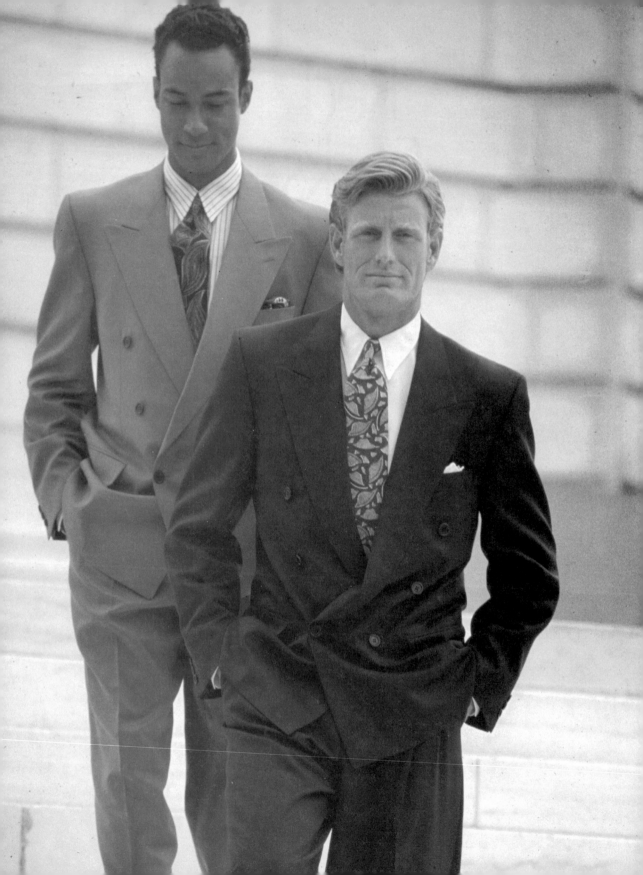

Red Socks Don't Work

✖ ✖ ✖ ✖ ✖ ✖

MESSAGES FROM THE REAL WORLD ABOUT MEN'S CLOTHING

✖ ✖ ✖ ✖ ✖ ✖

KENNETH J. KARPINSKI

IMPACT PUBLICATIONS

Manassas Park, Virginia

Copyright © 1994 by Kenneth J. Karpinski

Illustrations © by Martha Vaughn

Cover and text design by Joyce C. Weston

Photography is courtesy of Britches of Georgetowne and
Joseph J. Pietrafesa Co. © Hal Silverman Studio

Necktie patterns and tie tying examples by Robert Talbott,
Talbott Studio in Carmel, California

Library of Congress Cataloguing-in-Publication Data
    Karpinski, Kenneth J., 1948-
    Red socks don't work: messages from the real world
       about men's clothing / Kenneth J. Karpinski.
    p. cm.
    Includes index.
    ISBN 1-57023-007-2 : $14.95
    1. Men's clothing. 2. Grooming for men. I. Title
TT618.K37 1993
646'.32--dc20   93-43382
                               CIP

For information on distribution or quantity discount
rates, Tel. 703/361-7300, Fax 703/335-9486, or write to:
Sales Department, IMPACT PUBLICATIONS,
9104-N Manassas Drive, Manassas Park, VA 22111-5211.

Distributed to the trade by National Book Network,
4720 Boston Way, Suite A, Lanham, MD 20706,
Tel. 301/459-8696 or 800/462-6420.

Acknowledgments

There are thirteen people without whom I could not have produced this book. They were enormously helpful and I want them all to know how much I appreciate their contributions.

First, I'd like to thank Judy, my wife, friend and the best partner anyone could be lucky enough to have, for her rock-solid faith, encouragement and support.

Pam Leigh helped most with her unfailing good humor and an incredible ability to make each and every word say exactly what I needed it to convey.

Ron and Caryl Krannich, my publishers, made this project an absolute joy. They have become very important to me and I look forward to working with them for many years to come.

Martha Vaughan's illustrations and Linda and Harriet Ripinsky's production work are the best I have ever seen. They were unfailingly professional and forgiving, even when my requests were beyond the realm of possibility. I consider them to be the best in the business.

For their thoughts, ideas and genuine concern, my heart-felt thanks to Pauline Barney and David Clubb.

They worked under impossible deadlines and yet never failed to offer their advice and wisdom, which I gratefully accepted.

David Pensky and Britches of Georgetowne became enthusiastic supporters from the moment they became involved, and that meant a lot to me. Photographs of Britches' clothing are found throughout.

Joey Pietrafesa and Ellison Crain of the Joseph J. Pietrafesa Company, two very classy people, in the truest sense of the words, helped to make this book a reality. Much of the clothing photographed came from them including the beautiful vicuna cashmere blazer on the cover.

Red Socks Don't Work evolved from hundreds of mentors and literally thousands of "Gentlemen" over a period of more than ten years. My sincere thanks to all of them for allowing me to learn from them and to bring these messages to others.

Contents

APPENDICES

Author's Note

When I first wrote *The Winner's Style*, I had been in the men's clothing industry for a respectable number of years and had earned a reputation for being able to "shut up, listen, and learn." So, the wisdom of many people was transmitted to the pages of Style and not just my own opinions, even though those were in no short supply. As the years went by, the thought of changing or updating the advice would come up from time to time. And, yet, when held up to scrutiny, very little about the original pages seemed to need alteration.

However, after nearly six years of conducting my "Personal Packaging Seminars" to a wide-range of audiences—high tech to no tech, State Department and Foreign Service Institute employees to local Jaycees and Rotary Clubs and college and university students—I learned that men still needed to learn the basics of clothing selection.

That men need this information was reinforced while spending more than five years working on the men's clothing floor at Nordstrom—considered by many as a leader among the men's clothing retailers today. During my time there, I helped a lot of men—doctors, lawyers, politicians, students, businessmen, salesmen, retiring military, graduates fresh out of school as well as the heads of some of the largest corporations in America. They were all good at what they did, and they seemed to appreciate that I was good at what I did as well.

Some of the same questions were asked over and over by young and old alike. There were many misconceptions and much misinformation. There was also important information they had never heard. Hence, all of the information that these men needed—plus the latest menswear knowledge—is included in this new edition.

I am truly grateful to all of those people who were willing to teach me a little of what they knew and, also, to my "gentlemen"—which is how I always referred to the many men I assisted personally over the years—for appreciating my knowing this stuff for them.

I have begun countless seminars with the following words and they seem very appropriate as we begin to share these messages from the real world: "MENSWEAR MOVES IN MILLIMETERS." Once you have the knowledge, it's yours for a long, long time.

Red Socks Don't Work

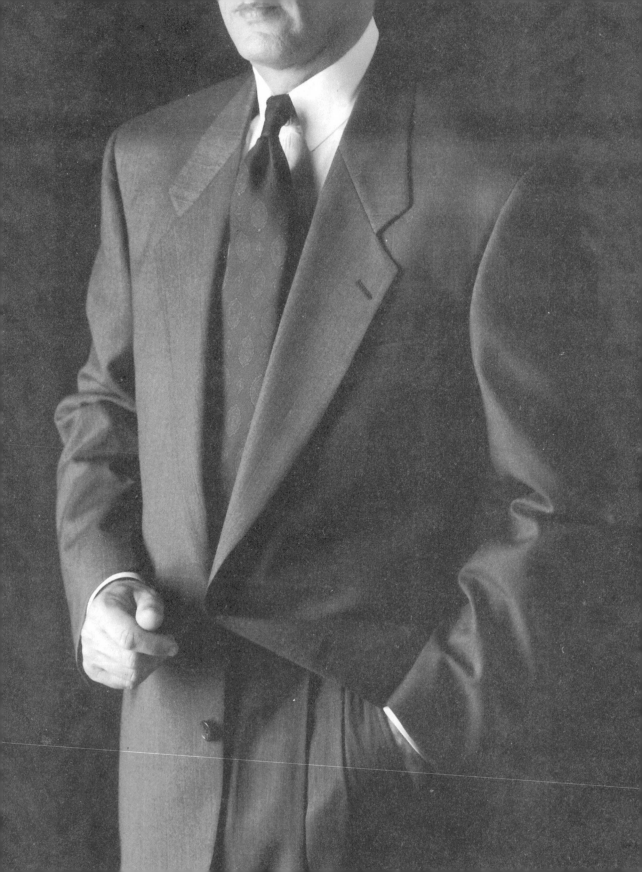

1 | Messages from the Real World

A long with dressing appropriately for the occasion, comes the undeniable need to look current. I'm not suggesting high-fashion, trendy, or exaggerated clothing, especially in the corporate or professional environment. It is just not acceptable. However, keeping up with the times is important. At the conclusion of my "Personal Packaging" seminars I show a slide of an advertisement from a well-known designer in a highly respected men's fashion magazine under the title of "Staying Current." The photograph never fails to cause an audible gasp from the group because it appeared in the 1972 edition of the magazine, and some of the group recognize themselves and realize they have not revamped their look since 1972.

Don't forget that other people form an opinion of you the first time they meet you, and that impression can take a long time to change. It's important, then, that the first meeting be positive and accurately reflect the inner you. It's certainly a lot simpler to make a great first impression with your appearance and then follow up by showing what a capable, impressive and trustworthy person you are performance-wise.

Occupation, age, position and what area of the country you live in will all contribute to what constitutes current but not outrageous fashion sense. In fields like advertising, television, consulting, public relations—areas that are considered to be artistic and creative—you have more flexibility with colors, designs, fabrics and patterns. It is not only appropriate but expected that you be on the cutting edge if you work in these fields. For the rest of us, it's important to understand the fashion direction and to reach for it slowly, according to your personality, age, the type of work you do or hope to do and the occasion.

For the purpose of illustration, we will examine a number of representative occupations and get the input of men who are currently very successful in them. Each will discuss what clothing works for their job and how to dress when interviewing for their occupation and to succeed once you are in it.

MEDICINE

According to Dr. Leonard Rosen, O.B., GYN., "People expect professionals in medicine to be neat and clean and to wear clothing that inspires confidence."

Doctors spend more of their working hours in a lab coat, smock or scrubs than in traditional business apparel. Many doctors tell me that they only wear a sports coat on the way to work and when they leave to go home, and that the only time they need a suit is for a business function, a social affair such as a wedding, Bar Mitzvah or funeral, or for a professional meeting such as a hospital board meeting. On these occasions the colors and patterns will lean more toward mid-blue, blue-gray, subtle plaids and solids and away from the more formal, serious patterns.

Assuming this is, indeed, the case with most doctors, their shirt and tie play a much more important role in the way they interact with others. Because of the stark nature of a white lab coat, a little color or pattern in the shirt is highly recommended. Blue, yellow, pink and virtually any stripe will add life to the outfit. By being a bit creative with the necktie, the doctor can create a mood to soothe, cheer up or provide a feeling of stability to his patients.

One of my gentlemen is a young physician who is one of the gentlest men I have ever known. He is also 6'4" and the head of a cancer treatment clinic. Because of his size and the nature of his practice, he finds it helpful to lighten the mood a little by wearing ties that are softer and less business-like such as paisley, floral and colors that are not too bright or shocking. Another doctor client spends much of his time as an administrator, with dozens of people seeking a piece of his time and counsel. For a long time we selected ties that were simple and conservative, but one day, on a lark, I pulled a fun conversational tie out of the case and asked if something fire engine red with a basketball player in mid-dunk would interest him. I wasn't surprised when he said no. What shocked me was when he asked, "How about the one with a fish being hooked by a fly-fisherman on it?" I literally gasped "Really"! He had decided that this would be his fun tie. "When I wear this tie to the hospital everyone will know that I'm in a good mood." (I have heard from staff members that word spreads quickly when the good doctor is wearing his fish tie.)

LEGAL

Richard Scalise, an attorney-at-law, suggests there are a few identifying features to the way lawyers, young and old, dress day in and day out: A dark suit, with or without stripes; braces (they send a strong message and make you feel more fully dressed when you remove your jacket in the office); white shirts, clean, fresh, lightly starched and with no signs of fraying; leather soled shoes and over-the-calf socks.

The one pet peeve that drives him to distraction is the area around the collar: "If you add up all the layers of fabric that a man wears around his neck it's a wonder anything ever gets done. If you include longish hair that reaches the collar there are FOURTEEN layers surrounding the average man's neck, which gives new meaning to the term ' hot under the collar.' "

Lightweight suit fabrics seem to be the overwhelming choice of attorneys who spend most of their time indoors with a jacket on. Solid colors and pinstripes occupy a large percentage of their closet space. Sports coats are reserved for social wear. The one deviation from the serious solid or pinstripe look is the non-court suit—where some attorneys who want variety and a dash of fashion will agree to try a plaid or earth-toned suit.

For the most part, the younger attorneys in a firm are quick to pick up what is acceptable by watching and wearing what the partners are wearing. Overt displays of individuality don't seem to be welcome in this environment. If in doubt, stick to the more serious looks. John Joseph Cassidy, Partner in a prominent, Washington, D.C. law firm, says, "First impressions are important because they are lasting impressions, and it does matter that attorneys are appropriately dressed whether they are meeting a client in their office or appearing in court."

POLITICS

"In politics," according to Congressman Mike Synar, from Oklahoma, "the first impression may be the only one you get. People in public service must wear quality clothing. People recognize it and they expect it. It is reassuring and it inspires confidence. In politics, the successful rely on the advice of experts in a number of areas: polling, law, public relations and research—to name just a few. Finding and using the advice of an image expert only makes sense."

Congressman Synar and I have worked together for a long time. One of the most thrilling calls I ever received was from him when *Roll Call Magazine* named him to their Best Dressed List. "Thanks pal, you made this happen," is all he said.

HOSPITALITY

People in the hospitality industry are in the public eye all day, every day. Many companies have decided upon uniforms to add to the ambience and eliminate gaffs in judgment. An excellent rule of thumb from image expert Joanne Nicholson, President of Color 1, an image consulting firm and author of *Color Wonderful* is this: "The higher the price of the room in your property the dressier you should look."

Fellow image expert Angie Michael, President of Image Resource Group, Inc., feels that approachability must be a top priority in the 90's. "In a large downtown hotel, a double-breasted suit may be right at home, providing patrons with a sense of security and confidence; however, a motel on an interstate highway or a motel or hotel in a small town may find its owner or manager in a sports coat and coordinated trouser—maybe even wearing a non-traditional dress shirt and a string tie around his neck."

TRANSITIONING MILITARY

According to William K. Suter, Major General, U.S. Army (Ret.), "When you are interviewed for a job, two appraisals are taking place. You and your clothing are being evaluated. When I retired and began the job search odyssey, the first thing I did was find a top flight clothing consultant to get me properly dressed. The expenditure was not small, but it was a rewarding and lasting investment."

General Suter adds that doubts, fears and a feeling of apprehension due to such a dramatic change—leaving the military family—leave a man in a very vulnerable position where he may accept help and advice from anyone willing to offer it and not necessarily from those informed enough to help him.

Lt. Colonel Greg Huckabee also has a number of insightful observations to offer the man transitioning out of the military into civilian careers: "Most of us in the military do not have a clue as to what is appropriate in the civilian business and professional community. This is because we never needed to know about suits and sports coats beyond the all-purpose ones we had in our closets for strictly civilian functions such as funerals, weddings and cocktail parties. Interestingly, younger Army lawyers seem to be the best equipped when making the transition since they still have the suits they wore while clerking in civilian law firms right after law school."

Colonel "Huck" thinks it all boils down to the years spent operating in a team atmosphere versus making an effort to "standout" for a civilian job. He remembers one military comrade that he sent to me who returned wearing a new interview suit. His pleased comrade said, "I feel like a different person; I have a feeling of confidence I didn't have before."

It is a game of competition; whether you get the job is really a matter of how you fit into the environment. You must accept the fact that everyone called in for an interview has an outstanding resume, and for you to be successful you must take advantage of the critical first few minutes of an interview—to look impressive and stand out from the crowd.

Martin Kaufman, recently retired from the U.S. Air Force and now a consultant, shares a fabulous bit of wisdom that worked extremely well for him: "In advance of making the change, find a store you like, learn when they hold their sales and buy one suit at a time to prepare. Three or four at one time can cause sticker shock."

✖ ✖ ✖

GOVERNMENT WORKER

Susan Drew Thomas is a career transition strategist for The Department of State's Career Transition Center. She advises: "Too many people spend a great deal of time preparing their resumes but only about half the time getting ready for the actual interview and even less than that when preparing their wardrobe. In reality all three phases should be given equal attention: a perfectly organized resume, flawlessly prepared; questions and answers carefully thought out and practiced until comfortable; and a dress rehearsal of what they are going to wear and having determined what image or message the clothing should convey."

Sadly, too many people have the following image in their minds when they think of a government worker: Someone who is wearing an out-of-date sports coat and tie; clothing indigenous to their last Third World tour of duty; a short-sleeved shirt, with pens in the front shirt pocket; and boxy, rubber-soled shoes. Also, the jacket is frequently off and the shirt sleeves, if long-sleeved, are rolled up since this is perceived to be the work uniform of a hard-working and sincere member of government service.

Susan has a few bits of advice for those trying to get in or be promoted within the government: 1) Get a long-sleeved shirt. 2) Make sure it is pressed and starched for the interview. 3) Buy a new tie. 4) Dress one step above where you now are or want to be.

ENTREPRENEUR

The single most erroneous myth many people have when going out on their own is that finally they can dress any way they want. Richard Kinnaird, Jr. founder of The Training Group, which provides high-end computer training for businesses, began his own computer software training company after working for many years at several very large corporate companies. When I asked him how his dressing habits had changed now that he's his own boss, the answer surprised me: "Now that I think about it, I'm more careful now than when I was an employee of a big name company. I realized that I am the company and credibility begins with me. When I am in front of my students I feel it is a matter of respect for them and a way to distinguish myself from my client. So I am always in a suit, if appropriate, or a blazer, tie and a pair of coordinated trousers."

After years of providing Rick with the white shirts he assured me he must have, the last time we worked together I suggested he experiment with some stripes to see how he liked them; now striped shirts are becoming a part of his sartorial signature.

Lisa Cunningham, an image expert and Adjunct Professor at Parson's School of Design in New York City, deals with a lot of men who are going out on their own. She says that she always asks one simple question and then offers one strong piece of advice: "Who are you going to try to work with—banks, Fortune 500 companies, doctors, lawyers or Indian chiefs? Once you decide that, dress according to the way they dress."

Geoffrey Lewis is President of the Lewis Enterprise Group (LEG-UP), and is one of the best dressed young men I have ever known. He says, "Don't kid yourself, you still have to dress the part. You have to compete with the 'Blue Chips' and must look as though you're up to it."

NON-PROFIT EXECUTIVE

It seems men who work for a non-profit organization are in a wonderful situation. They spend their days toiling for a cause that will produce a better world for all of us, and they get to dress like it is 'casual day' every day. It is true that a suit is often not needed or even proper in normal daily operations. One may be needed when meeting with executives from the outside, when appearing before a congressional committee or when traveling. For the most part, their wardrobe would consist of a good quality, well-fitting blazer or subtle sports coat; several color-coordinated or neutral trousers such as khaki or light olive; and a handful of shirts in denim, chambray, woven patterns and knit solids as well as a few traditional oxford cloth button-downs—all of which would be at home with an interesting conversational, cause-related tie, knit tie or even a string tie with a special slide.

Too serious a suit, even in those circumstances where a suit is called for, can look all wrong—the old "duck out of water" syndrome. Skip the super-serious pinstripes and try a solid navy, gray or earth tone depending on your personal color preference. They are not only easier to combine with a shirt and tie, they are understood by everybody and disliked by no one.

SALES

Kyeson Cummings works in high-end, real estate securities sales and offers a number of tips that he has observed on his way to becoming a leader in his industry:

"Suits should be the best you can comfortably afford. If you're dealing with ultra-successful people, they know the difference and feel more comfortable when working with peers, or at least those on the way up. Look good from head to toe, no detail will escape notice; take regional and industry differences into account when choosing the clothes to be worn on a sales call. In other words, dress with the individual with whom you will be working in mind."

Don Graling is an Account Executive in telecommunications solutions specializing in the Federal Government who deals with multi-million dollar contracts which may last five or more years. He finds that conservative credibility is essential to his success. "A dark blue suit, white shirt, black leather shoes and belt and really good ties are all important to creating an air of professional competence. And don't forget the shoe shine; your shoes must always be highly polished even if you have to do it yourself every day."

Some men in his company enjoy shopping more than others, but they share the expertise of one woman at a local department store who has gained their confidence by being able to select the perfect tie for each of them. As you might expect, the older, more successful of his colleagues spend considerably more for their clothing than the younger salesmen who are just starting out.

Salesmen have one universal challenge—looking up-to-date without looking slick and dressing to project a professional/high quality image without appearing aloof or unapproachable. Julian Brylawski is a sales training consultant who advises, "Clothes should be warm, professionally conservative and unobtrusive—that is, they should not attract too much attention. Because of the many different situations I find myself in, my overall goal is to make the prospect feel comfortable."

One area Julian feels strongly about is that clean, well-selected garments are more important than buying expensive names or fabrics and looking rumpled in them: "Having certain clothes that feel good and that you wear only on important sales calls or presentations is often-heard advice that I agree with wholeheartedly. Keep them clean, well-pressed and ready to go, and you will be amazed at how just putting them on can boost your self-confidence."

Investment advisor, Seabrook O. Shaffer says, "You can never have more than ONE first introduction. You must be dressed to meet the crowd or individual with whom you will be working. If you cannot afford expensive new suits, then get less expensive new suits to allow you to feel good about yourself and radiate confidence to others; be certain your hair is well-trimmed and your hands manicured; shoes are extremely important as finishing touches—people really do notice them and, when cared for, they help you exude an air of quiet self-confidence."

INTERVIEWING

According to Mark Albrecht, Vice-President, Human Resources, "Most of us take about two minutes to form an impression and then spend the next 30 minutes deciding if it was right or wrong. If the interview is the best possible impression you can make, why would you not go out of your way to be certain everything is as perfect as possible. You would not print a resume on loose leaf paper, so why would you present yourself with any less care?"

Expensive, designer clothes are absolutely not essential to getting a good job regardless of the industry. Most recruiters or personnel executives know that those just starting out are on limited budgets. But they all expect clean, appropriate clothing that fits with the style of the company where you are interviewing.

Career Counselor Barbara Cox Farris advises, "Dress conservatively and watch your grooming, they are both important. Wear clothing worn by those already in the profession or organization at levels you aspire to or hope to be considered for. Appearance makes a big difference. First impressions color the way people react to you for a long time."

Clothing Consultant Angie Michael has a rule of thumb that she shares with people in all walks of life to help them sort through the many new patterns of ties available today: "If the pattern on a tie represents something that moves or is alive—then it probably should be saved for non-business wear." Angie suggests the following guide to determine your tie's pattern size:

- If the size of the pattern is smaller than a quarter—almost always OK.
- If the size of the pattern is larger than a quarter but smaller than two—probably OK in more stylish situations.
- If the size of the pattern is larger than three quarters—it speaks too loudly and is beginning to be too expressive.

Also, Angie feels that those starting out in sales should be careful when wearing a double-breasted suit. She says, "It tends to be too formal and powerful in most situations. You must be seen as friendly and approachable."

Consultant Joanne Nicholson says, "Feel good about how you look all of the time—even if you are on the phone. It reflects on how successful you feel about yourself!"

FROM EAST TO WEST—NORTH TO SOUTH

The general codes of dress presented here are the most universally accepted. They apply no matter where you live or work. Of course, there are certain regional differences, but, for the most part, these are relatively minor. For example, in Southern California (in contrast to the northern regions of the state) there is some room for brighter hues, a more relaxed feel and a slightly more expressive style than you are likely to find in the northeast.

In Texas, suede jackets, or those with a trimmed yoke, are worn with boots as a matter of course. Only those who are born and bred in Texas can really pull this look off easily and with style. In Florida, where weather truly plays a role in the way a man dresses, lighter colors and fabrics are an accepted common sense solution. Obviously, it would be a mistake to wear Florida apparel for business in Chicago, Seattle, Boston or New York where time spent outdoors and the relative temperature call for much more substantial body covering. Don't try to second-guess regional differences from a distance. Chances are you'll guess wrong. Apply the universal code of quality and quiet good taste no matter where you are, and your appearance will never slow you down.

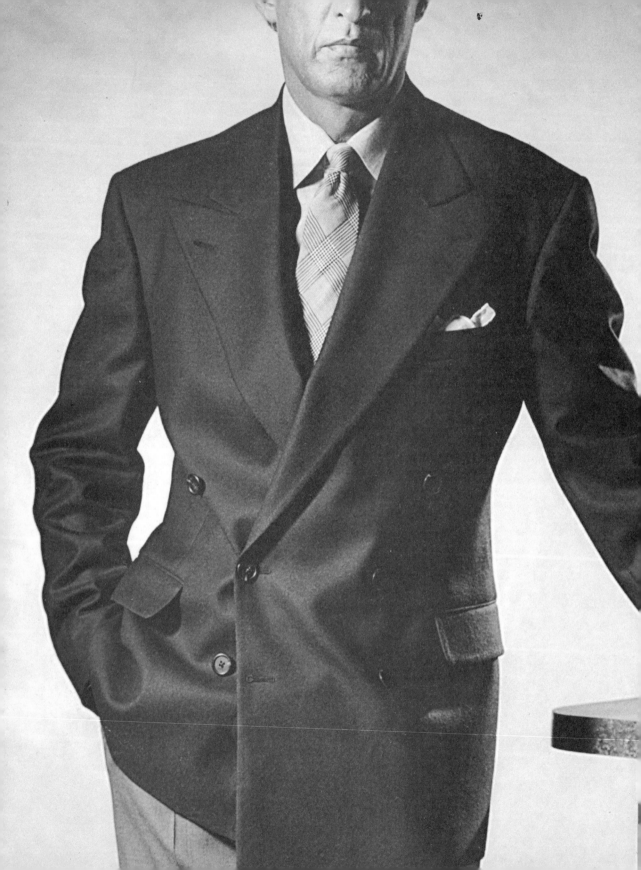

2 | Sharpening Your Persona: Importance of the "Right" Dress

There's a common misconception that men don't change very much as they grow older, hence the chestnut: "The difference between men and boys is the price of their toys!"

Indeed, this saying has a nice settled ring to it, a comfortable old shoe aura. If only it were true. The truth is that men do change, sometimes in radical ways. From boyhood to CEO, they must continually adjust to these changes and update their persona. If they fail to do so they are stuck in a rut, and this is a prelude to disaster in every facet of their lives. The psychology textbooks are filled with the ups and downs of male "passages," their changing needs for love, praise, recognition and money. There are hundreds of ways to accommodate these passages, but the one we are going to deal with here is the way in which men influence the way others relate to them—how the world "out there" sees them.

We've all heard the expression, "You can't judge a book by its cover." However, publishing houses have long since proven that covers may not tell you what's inside a book, but the cover is the reason that we pick up one or another off the rack. Until it is picked up, no sale is made.

Men are in the same position. And, to overcome resistance, they use the one tool that is at their disposal and completely under their personal control: outward appearance. This book is designed to help you use this "cover" to its greatest advantage.

Of course, there are changes in "cover," adjustments dictated by dozens of factors ranging from the physical to the professional. As we grow older or simply move through the various stages of our career, we need to adapt our outward appearance to project who and what we are. A major object of these changes is to present to the world the image of being a person who deserves to get the greatest rewards. While it is true we are all individuals, many of us pursue surprisingly similar goals. The categories most often mentioned are: 1) promotions; 2) more money; 3) new opportunities; 4) social acceptance; 5) trust and believability; and 6) confidence. If you seek any or all of these things, you're not alone. Here are the stories of a few men who have gone before you; learn from their experience.

CASE HISTORIES FROM THE REAL WORLD

Know Your Audience (The Cases of Walter W. and Dan R.)

It was 2:30 P.M. on a cool, crisp Sunday afternoon when I greeted Denis, a very prominent attorney and partner at a firm with over 100 names on the letterhead. We had worked together many times before and I must admit I always enjoyed his precise approach to everything he did. He noted each detail and generalizations did not satisfy him; he needed to know why, how and what to expect from every feature. Out of the blue, he asked if I would consider doing a seminar for his firm, more specifically, the associates at the firm. Since seminars are what I enjoy doing most, I said yes without hesitating. Denis put his hand on my shoulder and added quickly: "There is just one thing; the reason we need you is to get through to one particular young man, (Walter W.). Although everyone will enjoy and profit by your presentation, Walter stands to benefit most. He is one of the brightest, most promising people we have recruited in years and we have big plans for him; but, he wears red socks every day with everything, everywhere. Some of the senior partners refuse to allow him to go on client calls for fear he will alienate some of our older, conservative clients who are set in their ways and expect to see their legal counsel present themselves in a certain way. To put it simply, we are wasting a lot of highly paid talent because of those damn red socks. You have to find a way to make the point without picking him out of the group. Can you do it?" I was being called in as a hired gun to do the dirty work and make it entertaining as well! We scheduled a luncheon meeting for all of the associates in the partners' dining room where we were surrounded by portraits of the legal titans who had gone before them.

The presentation went exceptionally well, the question and answer period lasted 30 minutes after the structured talk ended.

Three days later, Denis called to report that I had done it! The red socks were gone, replaced with subtle patterns on a background of gray or navy. Unique, individual and yet not so loud as to call attention to themselves.

Walter has since made partner, and is considered one of the best-dressed members of the firm. Often he is held up as an example to new attorneys in the firm as a role model. I still remember Denis' thoughts on the whole mission some time later, "Something so small should not have made a difference, but it did. I'm grateful he was as smart as we all knew he was and picked up on the hint about socks you gave out at your seminar that day. He'll never know the debt he owes you."

He may not, but every time I think about Walter I feel very rich.

Dan R. can be referred to as a dentist to the stars. He has a very successful practice, an active social life rubbing shoulders with the rich and famous, and a fulfilling family life. When asked whether he considers a person's appearance very important, he replied, "When I was in dental school I thought it mattered not a bit, but a seemingly minor event changed my mind about that."

"My wife and I were invited to a barbecue. The invitation read: Dress: informal. The event was being given by a corporate president on a big farm. When we arrived along with our good friends, we observed the "farm" filled with several hundred guests. Every man on the grounds was wearing a sport coat, many with neckties. My best friend and I had on short-sleeved knit shirts and slacks (mine happened to be jeans). Ben, my friend, went to the back of his car, opened the trunk and pulled out a navy blazer, put it on and disappeared into the crowd. I felt like a fish out of water all evening. One woman even asked me to bring out another bag of ice, assuming I was with the catering service. It was one of the most uncomfortable times I can recall, and though I had anticipated making a lot of high-level contacts, I ended up spending three hours behind a bush with my wife, watching everyone else have a grand time."

Inspire Confidence in Your Potential Clients (The Case of Ron K.)

A nationally known sales trainer and customer of mine Ron K. who specializes in telephone marketing is quick to point out that, more often than not, telephone contact is only half the job: "Most people want to meet the people with whom they do business and the way you present yourself will greatly influence how others perceive your opinion of yourself and your company's attention to detail. What we are seeing is more and bigger companies paying attention to the way their sales and marketing staffs look when working with their clients. Actually, it's the little things like shoes, neckties, and briefcases that are helping create a successful professional image."

Two case reports that illustrate these points (The Cases of Bill B. and Carter H.)

Bill B. is a senior partner of a wide ranging investment firm. He is a very meticulous person in all aspects of his life and after an incident a few years ago believes that most people, despite what they say, do judge a "book" by its cover. Here's what happened. One of his "rookies" (a salesman still in his first year with the firm), came into his office very upset. He thought he had made his first big sale. For weeks, by phone and letter, he had been selling this heavy hitter client (one who can write a check drawn on his personal account for $150,000) on a program the company was raising funds for. But the morning he went in person to pick up the check, he found the client distant and somewhat preoccupied. After only a couple of minutes came the news, "I've changed my mind; I've decided not to invest in your program." He stood up and showed the young salesman out. In an effort to save the sale, Bill picked up the phone and dialed the near-client's private line to see what had happened. After a brief introduction, Bill asked if the client would explain his sudden change of mind.

The client replied: "Have you ever taken a look at him and would you hand him $150,000 of your money?"

Bill then took his first close look at the rookie. He confessed he could see exactly what the client was talking about. The rookie really was a mess. His eyeglasses had tape holding the frame together; his tie was food-stained; he looked rumpled and his shoes were in need of a shine. In short, he didn't project a credible or professional image. Bill brought a currently popular self-help book into the office the next day and told the rookie to "close the door to your office and don't come out until you've finished it." Then he showed him a check in the amount of the commission he would have earned had the sale been closed—nearly $12,000.

"This is how important the way you look is," Bill said. "Fix yourself up."

Five days later, Bill and the rookie came out of the formerly reluctant client's office with a check in the amount of $200,000. Hard evidence of the importance of a man's appearance.

Carter H. is Vice President of Operations of a rapidly growing consumer product company with offices around the world. He had just finished moving the company's headquarters to new, enlarged facilities, and needed proposals from several large waste removal firms. He reviewed three firms that seemed reasonably priced and set up appointments to meet with their representatives. The first two were just short of what he was looking for and so he decided to wait and see what No. 3 had to offer. As it turned out, No. 3 had everything he was hoping for in terms of service and financial arrangements. But when the rep came in, he couldn't believe his eyes.

"The guy was a walking disaster," says Carter. "He really looked like he had just posed for a 'don't let this happen to you' poster. From the top of his unkempt hair to the bottom of his well-worn heels, this fellow was a mess."

Carter has a fairly simple code of business dealings: "I only do business with people and companies I can respect and who respect me, as well."

Carter told the rep that while his company's proposal was superior to the others, he could not consider doing business with his firm. The prospect of having this man in his office on a fairly regular basis seemed unthinkable, and Carter figured if he was representative of the waste removal company as a whole, then the company must be pretty shoddy, too. And yet, the bid was good, very good. Under the pretense of scheduling a second appointment, Carter telephoned the sales manager of company three and brought up the subject of appearance in a not-too-subtle way.

Two days later, company three's salesman was back, beautifully dressed and impeccably groomed. Carter couldn't believe his eyes. He signed the contract on the spot; it was a deal worth nearly $10,000 to the young man, who has since gone from near the back of the pack to the No. 2 salesman in the company.

The 7/38/55 Percent Formula (The Case of Gary S.)

Gary S., an executive in his late thirties, believes he learned the importance of how a man dresses back in prep school. The fellows with whom he prepped came from a wide-range of backgrounds, both culturally and financially. The one element they all had in common was their school blazer. "Once you put on your blazer, you became an equal. People gave you the benefit of the doubt, got to know you as an individual." As he grew older, serving in the U.S. Air Force and then in the business world as a management trainee, he observed that people immediately formed opinions about those with whom they came in contact. This opinion was based on nothing more than the other person's appearance. He also said that at least a dozen times in recent years he has heard other senior executives say, "they just don't look right" when reviewing prospective employees. The rejected candidates may be well qualified, but they simply don't know how to put themselves together—dressing and grooming wise—in a business environment, so they lose out. To show you how important Gary S. thinks the subject of looking the part is, in his office is a paperweight inscribed with the following, credited to professor Albert Mehrabian: "To develop trust and believability, 7% is what you say, 38% is how you say it, and 55% is how you look."

Dress to Concentrate on Business (The Case of Casey G.)

"I never used to think much about it," recalled Casey G., a financial planning advisor, "but I've changed my mind. I worked with an expert who evaluated and cleaned out my closet and then we went shopping for replacements. I can now say I enjoy going shopping and I'm considerably more confident that I project a successful, prosperous image to my clients. In my business that's important. Let's put it this way," he says, "maybe it's just a coincidence, but this year I will earn more money than ever before in my life and my wife loves hearing other women's compliments on the way I look when we attend parties. One thing I am sure of, though, is I can concentrate on the business at hand when meeting a new client and not think about my image. I know it's first-rate."

A Sharp Image: The Ticket to Promotions (The Case of Randy M.)

A gentle voice on the telephone said, "Mr. Karpinski, my name is Randy and a friend of mine suggested you might help me select some clothing." The next morning at 10 A.M. I was shaking hands with a casually dressed young man who had traveled several hundred miles to shape up his professional image. In just a few minutes, I had the information I needed about Randy. He was a successful chemical engineer and happily married but he had recently attended an out-of-town conference with people of similar backgrounds and expertise. During several break out sessions where the conversations inevitably turned to personal "war" stories, Randy heard others talk about calling on their companies' major clients, and the presentations they were planning to give in the near future. Randy realized he had never been asked to do either!

Later the same day, he was asked to come to the podium to summarize the possible solutions to a workshop project representing his group. "It then hit me like the proverbial ton of bricks," Randy told me. "Here I was surrounded by guys I considered to be my peers, and I looked like a bum compared to them! No wonder I was never asked to leave the labs. To tell the truth, I felt uncomfortable and decided to do something about it, so here I am."

We selected a not-too-serious suit pattern in a great earth tone which flattered Randy's hair, skin and eye color, fit him, was well-accessorized with newly selected shirts, ties and so forth, and was within his budget. He returned a week later with his wife who was thrilled with the transformation. "I've been trying to get him to do this forever," she confided in me while Randy was changing. "Thanks for your help."

Randy now volunteers for professional seminars and symposiums and proudly represents himself and his company. As an added benefit, his wife thinks he has never looked so handsome!

A Super Success Story (The Case of Jackson C.)

I met Jackson at a seminar on business image sponsored by the company he was associated with at the time. The morning session consisted of a presentation called "Personal Packaging" which offered help for both men and women, covering subjects from head to toe; it was followed by a break out session for those men and women wanting individual advice on clothing they already owned and wore routinely in their jobs.

As I progressed through the men, I came to Jackson. A nicer man you would never meet—quiet, polite, intelligent and wanting very much to improve his outward business appearance. But there was one significant drawback to getting my help then and there: he had with him almost nothing in the way of clothing for me to critique. The ties he had were great—current, flattering and, for the most part, expensive; but, he had no suits or sport coats. And yet his occupation indicated that he must, at least, occasionally wear these items. So why didn't he have them?

Jackson was a large man who simply could not find clothing to fit him. He had been wearing one sport coat—a nice tan year-round seasonal, and that was it. When he contacted me later for a private consultation, he was badly in need of advice. Ready-to-wear was not going to be an option for Jackson; his size was significantly beyond the scope of even the largest clothing inventory's size range. "Custom" clothing was out of his budget. So, we decided on made-to-measure which is lower priced than custom and offers fast delivery. For starters, we ordered a couple of extremely conservative suit patterns and a blazer. Talk about a new man emerging from the store!

A few months later, Jackson was back, this time buying a patterned sport coat, dress pants and another less conservative suit. Then, as the months went by, a tuxedo for a cruise as well as a double-breasted dark green blazer and a double-breasted dressy suit. He was having such fun creating his business image, and, best of all, it was paying off for him. After having spent several years at the same job, all of a sudden he received a promotion, the first of many.

Both Jackson and his wife feel that the clothes and his resulting sharper image have been the deciding factor which got his career moving. Now there is no stopping him; he's a smart, capable man who dresses professionally and is reaping the rewards of his efforts and the investment in himself.

Emulate Your Teammates (The Case of Harold L.)

Harold never got anything less than A's when he was in school and preparing for a career in academia. He was sought after by all the prestigious universities for both his advanced degrees and his winning personality. But after nearly 20 years in academia, he was wooed away by private industry "for a lot more money and perks" than he had ever dreamed of. He was to be the technical part of a team calling on senior executives considering the purchase of the high-tech products his new company manufactured.

Less than one month into his new job, he found himself in the richly paneled, plush carpeted office of the "wunderkind" CEO. "Harold," he said, "you are a great guy, everyone likes you and you have a way of explaining complex subjects so that everyone can understand them without feeling dumb, and that is exactly why we hired you. But, you just don't look like part of the team. We need to spruce up your clothes so you will fit in. To show you how serious I am about this, there is a check waiting for you downstairs. Go to the store of your choice and get yourself some new work clothes." Far from being offended, Harold appreciated the vote of confidence. After buying several presentation suits, travel clothes and all the necessary finishing touches, he feels like he has been reborn. Instead of just getting dressed, he now "suits up" for the day ahead. The last time

I talked to him, he ended the conversation by saying, "This has really been fun. I never realized how important dressing correctly is."

Winning Interviews (The Case of Kevin F.)

Going on job interviews is always stressful. This is true no matter if you are looking for your first job fresh out of school, finding a new job after losing one or just networking with people who may know of an opening you'd consider. What makes it so stressful? Is it the resume, answers to tough interview questions, the way you present yourself (verbally and sartorially) or some combination of all of these?

Kevin is one person who has a very definite opinion. Here is what happened to him: It was 3:15 P.M. one Tuesday and Kevin had just arrived for his appointment with the sales manager of his city's most successful magazine to discuss a newly created advertising-space sales position. Although he'd not really been looking for a new job, this unexpected opportunity promised a substantial increase in income. The offices were classically elegant and the receptionist warm and friendly. He noticed three other people already in the waiting area and presumed they were competitors. One by one they were called in and after about 15 minutes escorted out again with a warm farewell and hearty handshake. Now it was his turn. Kevin had barely settled into the chair across from the interviewer when he was hit with a barrage of all the standard and not-so-standard questions. Kevin expertly handled them all: open ended, closed, probing and even reflective. Then, the sales manager shifted in his chair, changed his tone and said: "As you may have noticed, a number of other people were here interviewing for this position, and, to be honest, based on their resumes and the chats I've just had with each of them, they all could probably do the job I need done. But, quite frankly, you look like the man I'd like going out to call on our customers. They are all very successful and feel most comfortable when doing business with people who also look successful. "

Kevin accepted the job then and there, and within two years had doubled his income. To this day, when he is asked for advice on handling job interviews, he tells people to make certain they have the best, most impressive resume possible, practice answering the tough questions with ease and, most important, take all the time necessary to make certain they look the part for the position they are seeking to fill. Dress as if the job depends on it because it just might. It did for him.

THE IMPORTANCE OF LOOKING LIKE A WINNER

These case histories make the point with which we began this chapter: men change! In these cases, the changes led to getting what they wanted. By placing a fine gloss on their appearance they learned that getting what they want and need is often a matter of looking as though they deserve it. In short, think like a winner, act like a winner, dress like a winner and a lot of formerly "impossible" obstacles will vanish.

Real Questions for Real Men

✖ ✖ ✖

None of the men whose cases we just reviewed set out to not look their best. Often it is a matter of knowing what is and what is not acceptable or when faced with several options being able to choose the best considering the specific situation at hand. Knowledge is power and to an extent knowing what you don't know is powerful as well. The questions which follow are meant to measure your clothing and grooming IQ. Answer them now on a separate piece of paper—put the answers aside while you go through the book. All of the answers will be found in the pages coming up. A passing score is 15 out of 20.

Remember, the questions you get wrong or are not sure of are image busters waiting to happen, even if it is just one or two. If you cannot wait, the answers can be found in the back of the book.

1. Is your hair cut appropriately for your face shape?
2. Should YOU invest in a toupee?
3. Can tinted glasses be worn indoors?
4. How can you tell when your shirt collar is too tight?
5. Is your favorite suit jacket/blazer too long or too short?
6. Are cuffs or plain bottoms correct on dress trousers?
7. Are your trousers long enough to be proper?
8. When can you wear a belt and suspenders together?
9. How should the width of your tie and lapel compare?
10. Is the wide or narrow end of the necktie always longer?
11. What kind of buckle is preferred in business wear?
12. Which briefcase material is best: leather, vinyl, plastic, metal?

13. Are your socks long enough?

14. How do you tell when your shoe's heels need replacing?

15. The most important piece of equipment used in a manicure is?

16. What necktie knot style is correct for most shirt collar types?

17. The four rules of combining coat, shirt and tie are?

18. When are black socks not appropriate?

19. Four different ways to wear a pocket square are?

20. On a shirt, is a French or barrel cuff considered dressier?

✖ ✖ ✖

All knowledge is of some value.
There is nothing so minute or inconsiderable,
that I would not rather know it than not.

—Samuel Johnson
Boswell's *Life of Samuel Johnson*

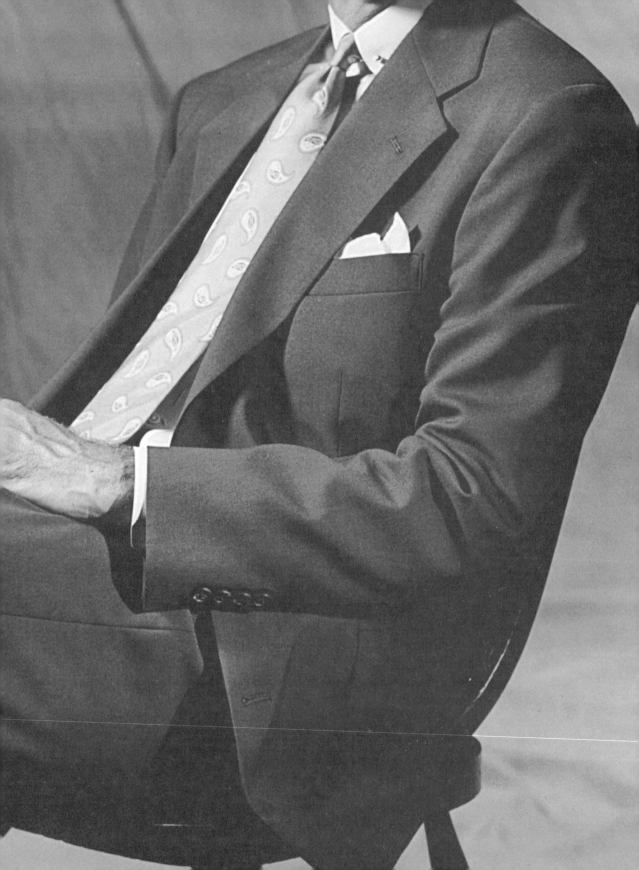

3 | Getting Down to Business: Your Suit

N o matter what your occupation, suits are an important part of your wardrobe for several reasons: they denote a seriousness of purpose and they say a lot about you; they are expensive; and they last a long time if properly cared for. So it is important to know the criteria for selection. Even men with a closet full of suits aren't necessarily in possession of a well-rounded suit wardrobe or the knowledge to create one.

After mastering this chapter—whether buying your first suit, or fine tuning your sartorial knowledge—you will walk into a men's clothing department or specialty store and be able to discuss your needs, wants and requirements with quiet confidence.

So, let's begin with patterns and colors, then move on to major styles, parts of a suit, shopping for a suit, fitting a suit—including common alteration marks—and finish with some notes on suits in general.

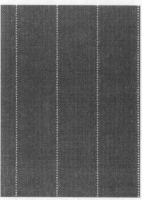

Pinstripes

PATTERNS

Pinstripe: A fine line either solid or broken (called a beaded pin) running vertically through the entire suit. Although usually in white or gray, you will also now see stripes of various colors—referred to as accent stripes—in addition to or instead of the basic white or gray stripe. The space between stripes

More Pinstripes

can range from one-sixteenth to one-and-a-half inches. As a general rule, the wider the spacing the dressier the pattern. Very narrowly spaced stripes can create an overly busy effect on a man with broad shoulders or who wears size 46 and up.

Chalk stripe: Stripes that are a bit wider resembling the lines drawn by a piece of chalk. This stripe is considered dressier and more conservative than pinstripes. Many men who are a little heavier labor under the mistaken idea that the wider stripes with an inch to an inch-and-a-half of dark fabric separating them makes them look even heavier. I have seen hundreds of men try on suits with chalk stripes and they all look elegant with the exception of maybe the very young. The wider spacing between stripes actually causes a slimming effect.

Herringbone: A ribbed, twilled fabric in which equal numbers of threads slant right and left forming a chevron-like pattern. This is a very beautiful pattern and is unfortunately absent from most men's closets. Part of the

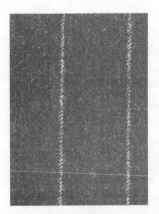

Chalk Stripe   *Herringbone*

reason is that this pattern is easier to make in slightly heavier fabrics not suitable for year-round wear. But as advances in manufacturing have taken place, lighter weights have been made available and now this dressy pattern (as long as it is subtle) is more easily found.

Plaid: Often called a glen plaid or glen check, it originated as a Scottish clan plaid. The box-like design, formed by groups of lines

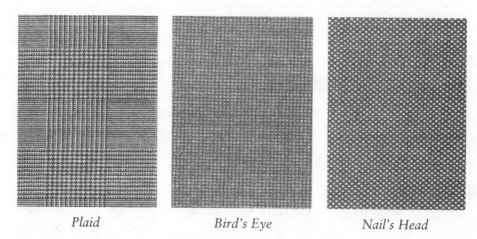

Plaid   *Bird's Eye*   *Nail's Head*

and houndstooth sections crossing at right angles, consists of black and white threads with an over-plaid in another shade or color. The formal, English name is Glen Urquhart from the clan of that name popularized by the Prince of Wales. Originally intended for country wear, it is now quite at home in the city for less dressy occasions and occupations.

Bird's Eye: A fabric with small, dark and light round dots resembling the eye of a bird. It is a less formal pattern very much at home in any business environment.

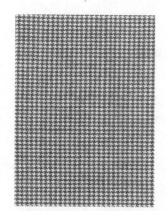

Nail's Head: A small dotted design used for sharkskin worsted in the United States. The appearance is that of a series of flat-head nails arranged side by side often slightly overlapping (also referred to as "pick-and-pick").

Houndstooth Check: A broken check that resembles a four-pointed star or the tooth of a dog. It ranges in size from micro in suits to large in sport coats.

Solid: The most popular pattern of all is no pattern. More solid color suits are sold to gentlemen across the country than any other single type. Colors are fairly limited to three major

Houndstooth

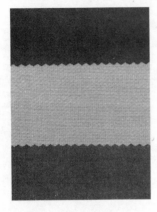

Solid

groupings: blue, gray and earth-toned. The beauty of these suits is their simplicity and ease of coordination with shirts and ties. Humble and unassuming on the hanger, a solid navy or gray suit can positively sparkle when paired with a good white shirt and well-tied tie. Accepted in any business situation anywhere in the world on anyone, young or old. I jokingly refer to these as my "no brainers" since no matter what I select to wear with them they seem to go together perfectly. Be a little careful with the earth-toned suits—the browns, olives, taupe and tans—they are less dressy but, depending on your individual hair, skin and eye coloring, can be very flattering.

COLOR

In the corporate world, there is not a lot of leeway in the color of the suit. Blue and gray suits are the accepted corporate colors, and are often considered "power suits"—strong, bold, yet quietly elegant. The darker tones give the wearer a firm presence without calling undue attention to any single element of the design.

Light and mid-tone colors can't be ruled out entirely. American style allows a certain amount of freedom, but the basic corporate wardrobe contains the standard blues and grays, almost exclusively.

STYLES: FINDING WHAT'S RIGHT FOR YOU

No matter if you're tall, short, thin, muscular, stocky or corpulent, most of the suits on the market today will work for you if the fit is right, and you have chosen the correct silhouette. For example, for many years it was mistakenly believed that only tall, thin men could successfully wear a double-breasted suit or jacket. Today this bromide is considered pure nonsense. If the silhouette and size are correct for the wearer, then the choice of a double-breasted model is an elegant option for any man who chooses to wear one. Many of the ready-made double-breasted suits hanging in the stores are referred to as a six-to-one. That is, there are six buttons on the front, but only the first or lowest button is meant to fasten. This button stance creates a long diagonal line that is very slimming and elongating—flattering to those who are heavier as well as those who thought they were too short to wear a double-breasted jacket.

By the way, if you're not sure which outside button to button on a double-breasted model, look for the anchor button to be fastened on the inside. These two buttons almost always correspond and should both be fastened.

The variety of suits on the market these days can be mind-boggling, but basically there are four kinds (with variations):

1. The "Natural Shoulder" Suit. Known as the "sack suit" when it was developed at the turn of the century, it is typical of American style and tailoring. It has a square front, unpadded shoulders, rolled lapels and pocket flaps. President Theodore Roosevelt wore this model, and it became the rage among those who wanted to emulate the Rough Rider's bold, broad-chested look. The first models had three or four buttons on the jacket; the three-button model won out because the lapels could be longer, giving the wearer a trim appearance. The jacket was slightly snug at the waist and hips.

It took a Democrat to change these details. President John Kennedy was a sworn two-button man, and Brooks Brothers, sensing a trend, came out with a twin-button version—this in the face of protests by some of Brooks' tailors and designers. It remains today as the traditional "ample cut" suit of classic American design.

2. The "European Cut". This suit has padded shoulders and fits snugly at the waist and hips. It is often seen with side vents on the jacket. The trousers have slightly flared cuffs. There are two- and three-button models. Its intent in design is to produce a slim, trim look by staying away from the traditional American full cut.

3. The "Updated Traditional American" cut is styled to reflect fashion trends. Depending on what's in, it may have side vents or a center vent. The shoulders may be padded and the jacket shaped to conform to

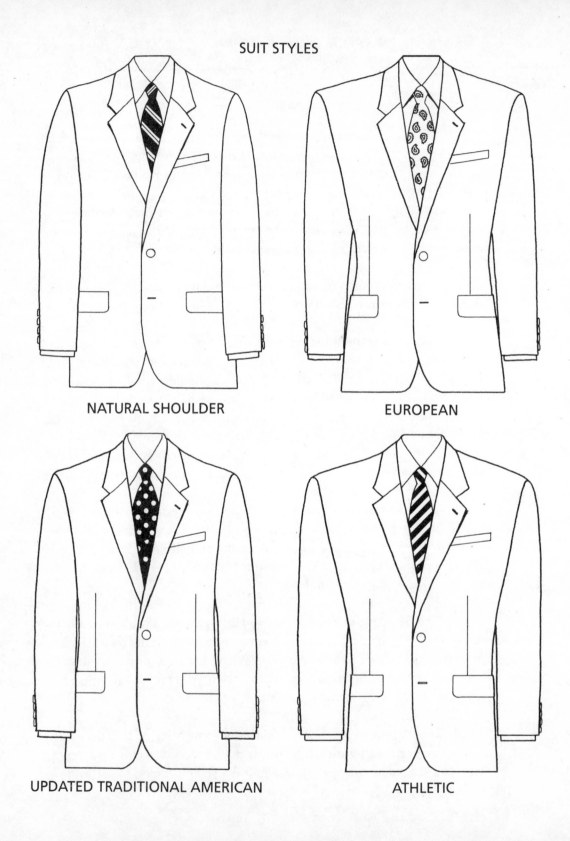

SUIT STYLES

NATURAL SHOULDER

EUROPEAN

UPDATED TRADITIONAL AMERICAN

ATHLETIC

fashion flows. The easiest way to look at this silhouette is to think of it as a mirror of current fashion that offers a certain amount of flair.

4. The "Athletic Cut" is becoming more popular, particularly on the west coast and to a lesser degree in the New York City area. This model has a drop from chest to waist of between eight and ten inches. Cut with larger shoulders and thighs, it is perfect for the swimmer or body builder who in the past had to have extensive alternations to obtain a proper fit.

None of these designs are cast in stone, however. Changes are constantly being introduced. What's important to keep in mind is that trendiness has no place in business. In the board rooms across America you are most likely to find the Updated Traditional American style and reasonable facsimiles. This is where appropriateness comes into play. The uniform has to fit the occasion, which is to say that you can wear any suit in its proper place.

A suit's silhouette and how it conforms to your body shape is more important than fabric, color, pattern or details despite what fashion experts have been espousing. If the silhouette is wrong, nothing, including alternation, is going to save you. So get this part right and all the rest is a plus.

Fit and appropriateness are the two unshakable rules. When it comes to the business of fitting suits to differently shaped bodies, fabric and fabric pattern count for more than anything else—after fit, of course.

A portly or stocky man should stay away from plaids, horizontal designs and heavy fabrics, such as tweed. These make him look broader. His best bets are wool blends, pinstripes and solid colors.

Very thin men do well with heavier fabrics and high visibility checks and other patterns. The patterns fill them out.

Muscular men also have to be cautious about patterns. Too much pattern in a suit can exaggerate their natural lines and make them appear ungainly. A properly tailored double-breasted model looks great on a well-built, healthy body.

✖ ✖ ✖

THE PARTS OF A SUIT

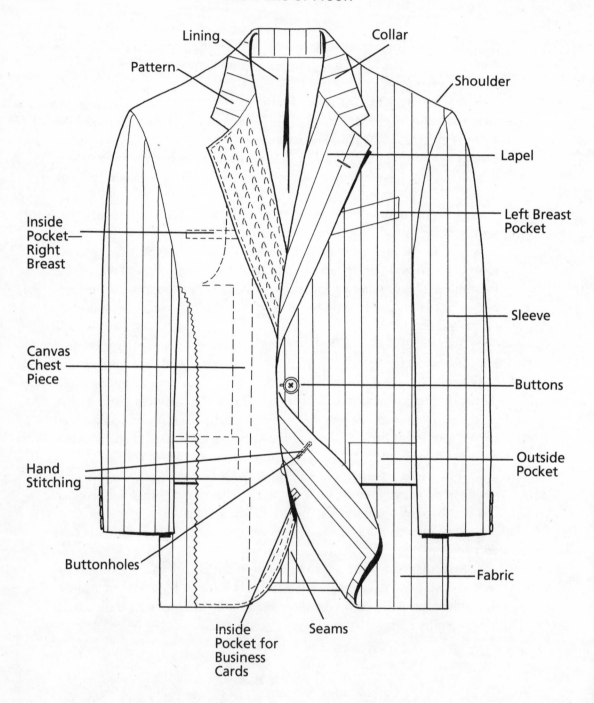

Lining

Collar

Pattern

Shoulder

Lapel

Inside Pocket—Right Breast

Left Breast Pocket

Canvas Chest Piece

Sleeve

Buttons

Hand Stitching

Outside Pocket

Buttonholes

Fabric

Inside Pocket for Business Cards

Seams

PARTS OF A SUIT: SIGNS OF QUALITY TAILORING

You don't need to know every detail of a suit to select and enjoy it for years to come. You do, however, need a cursory knowledge of some of the most important parts: what they are, where they are located and how they should work to your comfort and advantage.

Collar: Turn the collar up and look at its underside. There should be an under collar of felt or melton wool. In the best examples, the stitches should be attached by hand; the roundness that this allows will make the collar lie smooth and flat against the neck. (This is called anchoring and it is essential.) No space should be seen between the shirt and coat collar. If there is, something is wrong—the size, the fit, the style, your posture or any combination of these. A process called shortening the collar can correct some of this gapping, but it is difficult and expensive to achieve.

Canvas chest piece: Located in the front of the jacket, in the chest area, a piece of fabric is inserted between the lining and the outer fabric to give the jacket an even, smooth contour. The word fusing—heat-welding the chest piece to the fabric—used to be a dirty word; but now even some of the best made suits contain at least some. Softness is the essential key here; any stiffness should be suspect. The major danger of inexpensive fusibles is their tendency to break down in dry-cleaning, producing those unattractive "blisters" that can never be pressed away.

Sleeve: It should be set without puckering, "pitched" gently forward to hang cleanly and tapered slightly from the shoulder to the sleeves' hem. The lining will often be white, off-white or striped; industry-wide, one of the best is called Bemberg.

Body Lining: The jacket will be either fully or half lined depending upon the weight and stability of the suit fabric. Fully lined is not necessarily better. The lining color is usually but not always coordinated with the suit. The fabric often used is a Bemberg rayon which feels silky, is very durable, absorbs perspiration and allows the jacket to hang properly.

Seams: Look for clean edges with neat stitches. In a jacket without a full lining, the seams must be cut evenly, pressed flat and sewn smoothly to appear finished.

Buttons: Genuine horn, sewn on by hand and shanked (sitting on a little stem of fabric). Look for the cross-stitching through the button's holes.

Buttonholes: Hand-sewn and smooth on the outside, they may be rough on the inside. Durability is important here, since it is a stress point that is used over and over.

Pattern: Matching of patterns is essential in any well-made garment. It requires more fabric and more careful workmanship. Key points where the pattern should match are on the lapels, back seam, the pockets and seat of the pants.

Inside Pockets: There are at least three: a right and left inside breast pocket and a lower left inside pocket for cigarettes/business cards. All should be roomy enough to hold needed items.

Outside Pockets: There should be three: left breast and right and left side pockets. All should be lined in sturdy cotton to withstand constant loading of cargo. A nice touch in the right side pocket is a small inner pocket to hold change and keys. If yours doesn't have one, it can be added by your tailor.

Lapel: Lies perfectly flat against the chest without buckling or bowing out. To my eye the best looking edges are called "bluffed"—that is, no stitching is visible.

Fabric: It should be soft and pliant to the touch. Wool is the most desirable suit fabric; the higher the thread count (90's, 100's, Super 100), the finer the wool. No longer is wool uncomfortable for warm weather wear; tropical weight wools are cooler and more comfortable than almost any blend. Aside from the comfort, they also absorb dyes very well creating some of the most beautiful and subtle patterns ever seen.

Shoulder: An important element in the suit's style, very little if anything can be done to change the shoulder's expression. It is an integral part of the design. If it doesn't suit you, try another model. Look for smoothness and a clean line falling from the upper shoulder seam through the sleeve.

Hand Stitching: This is the second largest contributor to the cost of a suit. The more hand stitches per inch, the better the quality of the tailoring. The collar, sleeve, stress-points and buttonholes are areas that benefit from hand stitching.

✖ ✖ ✖

SHOPPING FOR A SUIT

You like the pattern and color, the cost seems to fit your budget, you've looked at the quality checks and feel comfortable that it is well-constructed, now on to the next steps:

1. Wear (or bring with you) appropriate clothes to visualize the final effect—the business shoes, shirt, socks and belt you would wear with a suit. If you haven't worn these items, see if they are available for you to use while trying on and fitting.
2. If deciding between two or more suits, compare the fit. Be aware that different models of the same maker may fit differently, so try all of them on even though you think you know how a particular maker's suits fit you.
3. Look at yourself in a three-way mirror. Turn to your right about 45 degrees and you should be able to see the back without twisting at the waist.
4. Check the jacket collar for "anchoring" (fitting flush with the shirt's collar—no gaps).
5. Button the top front button on a two-button suit. Minor pulls or horizontal creases can be fixed by the tailor.
6. Move your arms forward as if reaching. The small amount of extra fabric under your shoulder blades should allow for comfortable movement. The extra fullness under the arms is there for the same reason you have wrinkles on your knuckles, so you can bend them.
7. Sleeve length can be adjusted up and down within reason.
8. The lapels should lay flat or at least follow the contour of your chest. If you intend to carry a wallet or pocket calendar, put it in the pocket to see if the tailor will have a fighting chance of accommodating it.

 ## FITTING A SUIT

No matter how beautifully the color of a suit compliments your personal coloring, or how fabulous the "hand" (how it feels to the touch) of the fabric, you can't achieve an overall good look if the garment is improperly fitted.

You don't need to become a tailor to ensure your next suit fits you properly. Most good stores employ competent people to measure and fit you. But you still need to understand what you are looking at when you gaze into that three-way mirror so you can communicate with the man with the tape measure around his neck—or pins in his mouth.

Here is an easy-to-follow set of guidelines to allow you to feel confident while being fitted:

- The collar of the jacket should hug the back of your neck. If there is any space, it must be corrected. Also, if you see a horizontal bubble of fabric just below the collar between your shoulder blades, it should be eliminated by lowering the collar.
- The back of the jacket should fall smoothly and follow the curve of your back with no vertical creases. Depending on the fabric and pattern, the center seam can be let out or taken in.
- The vent (or vents) in the back should not pull open when you are standing erect. When considering a ventless model, be very honest with yourself. You must be fairly slim in the hips and not over endowed in the rear.

Whatever model you are considering—ventless, single-vent or double-vented (also referred to as side-vented)—the seat of your trousers should be covered.

- The waist of the jacket should conform to your own waistline. Only minor adjustments can be made here. If it hugs you too tightly or droops over you like a potato sack, you need a different cut of suit.
- Your shoulders should not bulge out past the sleeve head (that is the point where the sleeve is attached to the jacket shoulder); what you should see is a smooth line, from the shoulder all the way down the sleeve. Most men have one shoulder higher than the other. This can be evened out by inserting a pad in the lower shoulder.
- The front of the jacket should lie flat across your chest. When buttoned, the jacket lapels should lie smoothly, with no bowing out. If there is more than one finger's space between the lapel and your chest, try the next size or another model.

- It's important to check the alignment of the jacket buttons. Check to see if the bottom of the jacket lines up when it is buttoned.
- The correct sleeve length is the point where the hand meets the wrist. Simple. Be aware of two things when having this measured:

  1. Have both arms measured; believe it or not, most people have one arm longer than the other.
  2. Wear a long-sleeved shirt you would normally wear with a suit when being fitted. One-half-inch of shirt cuff (sometimes referred to as "linen") should show beneath the jacket sleeve.

- Make sure that your trouser creases are clearly visible from the bottom portion of the side pocket opening all the way down. If you see any horizontal lines at the waist, thigh, or knee areas, the pant legs are too tight and should be let out.
- The fit of the trouser waistband is important to your comfort. When trying on a pair of trousers, put your belt on and adjust it to see how you feel. If you wear braces, put them on and allow a little room for the trousers to hang properly.
- The break of a pant leg at the bottom depends on the height of the heel of your shoe. When being fitted, wear your business shoes—not your sneakers.
- When purchasing a three-piece suit, button the vest and tighten the belt at the back so that it feels comfortable. Then sit down and check the feel. Remember, when wearing a three-piece suit you will be removing the jacket but not the vest. Make absolutely sure the vest is comfortable and non-constricting .
- If you're active in your suits or have a job in which you move around a lot—for example, if you give presentations—be sure to try these motions at the clothier's. Tailors will usually fit you standing still. So move, bend, twist—and make sure the suit does the same, comfortably.
- Most of today's suits don't have "top stitching"—zig-zag stitching on the outside which is, in fact, the designer's "signature." However, you may find it on some European-made suits. It can be removed

safely without the suit falling apart. Of course, it's best to let the tailor handle it.

• If you carry your wallet in your inside pocket, place it in the pocket when being fitted. This allows the tailor to adjust for the extra room that will be needed to accommodate it. Do the same for the pants if you keep your wallet in your back pocket.

A NOTE ON EXTENDED SHOULDERS AND CLOSED VENTS

Two of the most recent innovations in men's clothing are the extended shoulder and the closed vent in the back of the jacket.

The shoulder is only a very small amount broader than in the past, but it adds a degree of comfort that many men find agreeable. By design it also adds a bit of extra drape to the back near the shoulder blades and possibly a slight fold of fabric in the chest area. This is part of the design and cannot be tailored out.

The vent has been around for a long time and men are used to seeing it. It spreads when we sit and when we insert our hands into our trouser pockets, it allows for easier access. The new ventless model creates a sleek, trim and very flattering line to the jacket because of the accentuation of the difference between the broader shoulder and the trimmer ventless back. Men with small, rounded shoulders should avoid them, as the suit's shoulder normally is too large for them and creates an out-of-proportion appearance. Young, well-built men generally look better wearing them.

At all stages of the fitting—as well as in the selection process—keep in mind Beau Brummell's advice. He said if a person turns to observe your dress, your clothes are "too new, too tight or too fashionable."

NOTES ON SUITS IN GENERAL

Here are two basic questions men have raised at my seminars:

#1. Are three-piece suits "out"?

Basically, the answer is no. Three-piece suits have been an accepted "uniform" for decades. However, as the price of fabric and construction climbed, stores tended to carry more two-piece than three-piece suits in order to cater to the economic needs of their customers. By eliminating the vest and encouraging two-piece suit sales, they were able to stay at a price range acceptable to the general public. The bottom line? It is A-OK to go for that three-piece suit if you can find it! Don't give up the right to decide for yourself if that is the suit that will help you find your winner's style.

#2. Are fully lined suits the ultimate sign of high quality?

For years, salesmen have been telling customers that "full-lined" was an indication of quality. Initially this was true. For example, winter garments made with very fine heavyweight piece goods had a full lining to add an additional layer of protection from the cold as well as to help the jacket slide on and off easily, and to lay smoothly on the shoulders. However, summer suits made of lighter weight fabrics had only half linings, since the extra protection wasn't needed. This did not make them necessarily any lesser quality.

Interestingly enough, some makers of mass market goods found that it was actually easier to put in a full lining and in so doing they could hide compromised construction. So a full lining doesn't automatically mean a suit is first-rate—nor does lack of a lining mean lesser quality.

BACK TO THE FITTING AREA—A CHECK LIST

When you return to the store to pick up your clothing take the extra time to be certain everything is the way you want it

Try on all of the pieces of clothing, take the altered one or ones back to the changing rooms where the fitting area is. Once you get that far, you have a good idea of whether or not your choices fit. Don't expect miracles; they don't happen in tailoring. If a change is promised, hold them to it! No change = no purchase.

Look at the following areas from top to bottom and follow along as the tailor checks the garment over:

1. **The Collar:** Most horizontal ridges or bubbles of fabric can be removed by lowering the collar.

2. **Shoulders:** Most men have one shoulder higher than the other. This can be evened out by inserting a pad in the lower shoulder.

3. **Blades:** Slight amount of extra fabric to allow for movement of the arms. A small amount must be present just behind the arms.

4. **Sides:** Can be taken in or let out to conform to your shape and preference.

5. **Jacket Length:** Should cover your seat completely. The center button should fall at about your navel. Because of pockets and overall proportion very little can be done here without destroying the balance.

6. **Vent:** Should lie flat and closed. If you carry a wallet in your back pocket, put it in there so the tailor can make any adjustments necessary for a smooth look.

7. **Sleeves:** Adjust to the point where your hand meets your wrist allowing a quarter to one-half inch of shirt to show. Be sure to have both sleeves marked. Almost everyone has one arm longer than the other.

8. **Trouser Waist:** Dress trousers should fit at the waist, not on the hips the way jeans or casual pants do. Most makers put up to two inches of fabric in the waist seam to allow for letting out.

9. **Seat and Thigh:** Can be let out or taken in to add room or get rid of fullness. Be certain the pockets are not gaping open or pulling; they should lie flat.

10. **Bottoms:** Trouser bottoms must break at the shoe tops. If you must err, do it on the side of being a little too long.

COVERING YOUR AMERICAN BODY WITH EUROPEAN CLOTHES

As with everything else, the rules for determining how the European sizing system translates into American body types seem to be made to be broken, so your safest bet is the most obvious: try it on first. The following guides, though, should help put you in the ballpark.

Shirt Sizes (inches/centimeters)

US	14in.	14.5	15	15.5	16	16.5	17	17.5	18
Europe	36cm	37	38	39	40	41	42	43	44

Sweaters/Sportswear

	small			*medium*			*large*	
US	38	40		42	44		46	48
Great Britain	38	40		42	44		46	48
France	44	44/46		48/50	50/52		54	
Italy	48	50		52	54			

Shoes

US	7	7.5	8	8.5	9	9.5	10	10.5	11	11.5
Britain	5.5	6	6.5	7	7.5	8	8.5	9	9.5	10
Continent	40.5	41	41.5	42	42.5	43	44	44.5	45	45.5

Made in U.S.A.

Pietrafesa

4 | Homing In on the Details

Now that you've learned the basics, it's time to focus on those make-it-or-break-it details of fit, fabric and style. Before I go on, however, I want to mention the importance of a woman's eye in this rather tricky business. The woman (or women) in your life has a keen sense of what works in a man's wardrobe. After all, your mother was probably the first person to dress you, and subsequent females, including wives and sisters, have continued the line of succession. While it's important to develop your own eye and sense of taste, the woman's "feel" in these matters can be more than a little helpful. It may be a good idea, too, to lend this book to the women in your life. Their critical appraisal can really pay off and save you a lot of unnecessary aggravation.

HERE, NOW, ARE THE CRITICAL CHECKPOINTS

✖✖ TOO SMALL—THE UNFORGIVABLE, UNBUTTONABLE LOOK

All too often your weight, or should I say your overweight, is the reason for looking poorly dressed. If you button your suit jacket or sport coat and the lapels do not lay flat against your chest, but bow out away from you, then your jacket is probably too small. If you can't button it at all, then it most certainly is time to move up and buy a larger size (seven pounds convert to one inch in size). Don't try to convince yourself that you're going to lose weight and in 30 days this 40 Regular will fit perfectly. All too often, men don't lose the weight. Better to buy the 41 or 42 Regular; and, if you do trim down, have it taken in—or reward yourself by hanging it in your closet to remind you how great you look when you're trim!

✖✖ PIPING AROUND JACKET AND LAPEL EDGES

I cannot think of a single reason for anyone to own a jacket with contrasting color around its edges or lapels. A little research suggests that the origin for this fashion detail was the colored stripes or bands on ancient Roman garments, which were used to denote rank. But it isn't acceptable in today's business environment. To be perfectly honest, it doesn't work in many social circles, either. It says cheap.

The one exception is a western-style sport coat of wool or wool-blend, edged in a very subtle shade of genuine leather, complimenting rather than contrasting the color of the jacket. You need to be careful not to abuse this exception. While it is a look much more at home at a casual outdoor affair, some parts of the country do allow it to be worn in business settings that are not too formal.

✖✖ DATED LAPEL WIDTH

Several years ago a group of men's clothing manufacturers decided to give men a reason to shop for suits more often. They reasoned that if they adjusted the width of the lapel every year or so, men would have to replace their clothing more often or else look badly dressed.

The effort was an unmitigated disaster, and you can rest assured that the width of men's suit lapels won't vary too much from the three to three-and-one-half inches now seen on most men's clothing.

Of course, as with any rule, there are exceptions. A few designers are working in slightly narrower lapels. Accessorized with the correctly proportioned shirt and tie, it is a very nice look.

A fairly safe rule of thumb for any situation is to wear a lapel width that is very close to half the distance from the inside of the lapel to the shoulder. You can't go wrong.

✖✖ FUSED CHEST PIECE

For a jacket or suit coat to hold its shape, it must have what is called a "chest piece." Generally this is made of coarse fabric and fits between the outer fabric and the lining. It is held in place in one of two ways. First, it can be fused, which means glued. This is the less expensive method, which has several drawbacks. It produces a very stiff front panel that doesn't conform to your body's movements. Also, except for the highest quality, the glue has a tendency to melt at high temperatures. So after a couple of trips to the dry cleaners, the front of your jacket will sprout small blisters of fabric. Currently, there is no way of repairing this damage.

Second, a manufacturer can sew in the chest piece. This is most often done by hand and is therefore a rather expensive process. This produces what is referred to as a "floating chest piece." The advantage to you is a very soft, springy jacket front that keeps its shape, moves when you do and won't be hurt by frequent dry-cleanings.

The bottom line: Avoid having your jacket stand up before you do.

✖✖ GANGSTER-WIDTH PINSTRIPES

Men's suits exist in solid colors, patterns such as herringbone, tic weave, plaids and pinstripes. By far the preferred uniform of American business men is the pinstripe suit. While it is very difficult to go wrong with many of the various types of stripes, it can be done.

Basic pinstripes differ because they are either formed by a series of beads or by a chain link pattern, or they have different space between the stripes. These spaces range from one-sixteenth-inch to as wide as one inch. Candy stripes are a fairly recent trend and use a colored thread such as blue, red or yellow instead of white to form the pinstripe. As long as the effect is subtle, "candies" can liven up your wardrobe, yet remain businesslike. Chalk stripes are also found in quality clothing. The effect is similar to the line that is created by a tailor's chalk on the fabric, and, for the most part, they are very subdued and sophisticated. However, you can get into trouble if the chalk stripe is too wide or in too much contrast with the suit color.

The rule is, if you can see that it is a stripe from across the room, be careful! The width, contrast or spacing may be too extreme for business use.

✖ ✖ ✖

✖✖ UNMATCHED PATTERN AT SEAMS

One of the most time-consuming and expensive features that can be very easily seen by the average shopper is how carefully the pattern (whether stripe, herringbone or plaid) is matched at the seams. The finest products will have a virtual mirror image at any point that two pieces of fabric are sewn together.

If you were only to check a few of the most important points, check the back seam, the lapels and the collar. From a distance this may not be a very noticeable point; but, up close, it is obvious.

The simple reason that more manufacturers don't do it is expense. To lay out all the pieces of a pattern by hand is a very time-consuming task that naturally adds to the labor cost. In addition, it means a waste of a great deal of fabric. At between $40 and $100 per yard for fine piece goods, this will add to the cost.

Many mass-produced lines use a computer to lay out a pattern so that virtually no fabric is wasted. That only helps the maker; it's no advantage to you unless the savings are passed on. I'm afraid we have not reached that phase yet.

✖✖ COLLAR NOT FITTING SNUGLY

Nothing can ruin the look of a suit or sport coat faster than an ill-fitting collar. If you put on your jacket and the collar doesn't lay flat against your shirt collar, exposing about one-half-inch of shirt, your jacket's collar needs to be adjusted.

This is very easy alteration for a qualified tailor. A precaution: Some less expensive suits do not have a hand set collar making it a bit more difficult for a tailor to reattach the collar perfectly. All the more reason to buy the highest quality clothing you can afford.

Another fit problem around the collar area to look out for is a "bubble" of fabric just below the collar of the jacket usually centered on the back seam. It can be avoided and, once again, any qualified tailor can correct it quickly and economically.

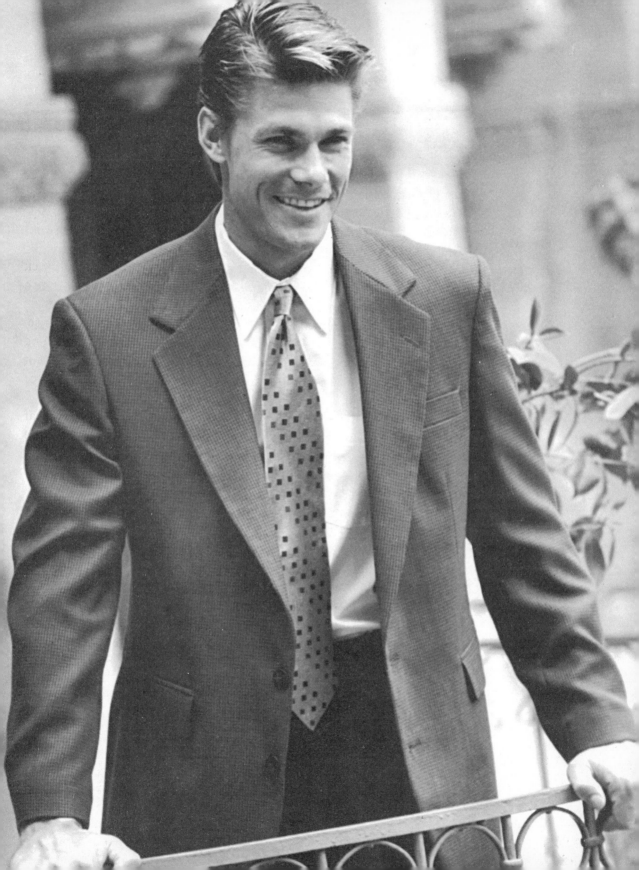

✖✖ PLASTIC BUTTONS

Believe it or not, most of the buttons on a man's suit or sport coat are not there to work. They are for decorative or historical reasons only.

One particularly fine suit maker is a fellow named Warren K. Cook. The firm that bears his name produces one of the better makes of suits available in Canada with limited distribution in the U.S. He has replaced the three or four buttons on the jacket sleeve with what is referred to as the "Cook Shield." This is an enameled "button" with the family crest emblazoned on it. To my knowledge, it is unique.

Manufacturers tend to use plastic to replace the bone buttons found on the finest of suits. I think this is an economical measure not in the customer's best interest as plastic buttons tend to break more often than bone.

✖✖ GAP-OSIS

Gap-osis is the condition that exists when a man's vest does not come down far enough to cover his belt line, and a line of shirt fabric shows through between the vest and the pants. The most prevalent cause of gap-osis: extra poundage that seeks out the upper body. The vest is meant to be snug fitting, but not that snug.

Now don't try to fool yourself. Don't stand in front of the mirror, suck in your gut, pull up your chest, pull down your vest, pull up your pants, and proudly declare that all is well. Stand relaxed with the bottom button open (some hefty monarch is said to have decreed this and you know how we are about following orders). If any of your shirt is peeking out, be assured that it is going to get worse after sitting and getting up a few times. There is no way to camouflage this situation, and the best advice is don't wear the vest until or unless it fits properly.

✖✖ MAN-MADE FABRICS

Remember when "polyester" denoted bad taste and poor quality? Fortunately, the polyester of today is vastly improved from the original.

Due to advances in technology, most of the disadvantages that existed, such as stretching, bagging and snagging, have been minimized or eliminated altogether. Polyester can now be spun, patterned and woven to resemble wool. It also can be woven together with natural fibers to create a soft, resilient and practical blend. When added to an equal or greater number of natural fibers (wool or cotton), it creates a garment that stays neat and crisp and even has a degree of breathability (though not as much as a 100% natural fabric). It is unarguably superior in terms of upkeep and in keeping its shape throughout a long plane flight or on a steamy day in the city.

One area where man-made fabrics still fall short is the way they take colors in the dying process. With most suit and sport coat colors this doesn't seem to be a problem, but be careful if you are looking for richness and depth of color other than a basic navy, gray or brown.

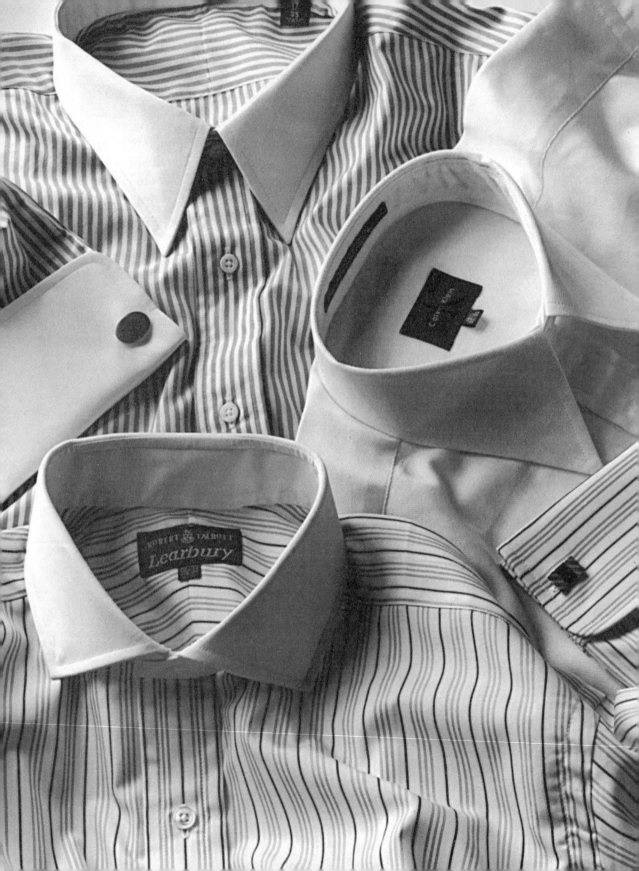

5 | The Shirt on Your Back

Far from being a mundane piece of body covering—which is how it began its evolution—the shirt has become a marvelous accompaniment to a well chosen suit. The colors, patterns and collar styles available today seem endless—certainly more than enough variety to suit the most discriminating male with acres of closet space.

Because it frames your face and is in such stark contrast to your jacket, everything about your shirt is very important. Fit, care and selection all come into play when it comes to this piece of clothing. Seemingly small mistakes take on great significance when they have to do with your shirt, so don't make the mistake of thinking that a mistake is so minor no one will notice. Make no compromises on this item of apparel.

Style and appropriateness, of course, are the most important criteria for selection, but certainly occupation, age and personal preference will influence the choices made.

But having said all that, one thing remains constant: Putting on a freshly laundered and pressed shirt feels wonderful! It doesn't matter whether you have one or one hundred shirts, every time you slip your arm into that pristine sleeve, everyday annoyances evaporate. It is the exact same feeling experienced the first time you were getting ready for that big holiday party or wedding or Bar Mitzvah or whatever. It doesn't change!

So, the next time you reach for that carefully folded or neatly hung shirt, no matter if it was professionally laundered or done at home with loving attention, remember all the special events in your life that called for a new shirt or a "clean, crisp" shirt and how it was always there for you, announcing to the world that you understood the significance of the day and were ready to meet the challenge.

Before we march out of our homes in triumph, though, let's examine the basic elements of a long-sleeved shirt—the collar, the cuffs, the fabric and the fit. We'll also include some common annoyances that can sabotage even the most well-dressed man.

COLLAR

There are many variations on the major shirt collar styles, but understanding a little about the most popular types can help you select the appropriate collar for the occasion:

The Button-Down Collar: This collar type is soft and is meant to have a slight inward or outward roll to it depending on the shirt maker. Of the two, I usually prefer the inward roll. It flatters most men and it is certainly the most comfortable collar style— and the most casual. It is correctly worn with blazers, sports coats, summer time cottons and blends, as well as year-round woolens. Be careful when trying to pair this collar style with a very dressy pattern or fabric as it can look out of place.

The Wide-Spread Collar: This collar is the most formal of all collar styles. This collar looks best with double-breasted jackets because the lines of the collar compliment the crossing lines of the lapels. You will often see this style collar worn with single-breasted jackets, but it would be incorrect to pair it with a blazer, sports coat or an informal suit. Caution: I don't suggest that men with thick, muscular necks or rounded face shapes wear it since it tends to exaggerate rather than flatter these features.

The Tab Collar: This collar is one of my favorites. It holds the tie in place by using tabs of fabric attached to the collar and held together under the knot of the necktie by means of a snap-tab, a button or a removable stud. The snap-tab is the easiest of the three closures to fasten and, therefore, the one to choose if you have to manipulate this before your first cup of coffee in the morning. This collar holds the tie in place very precisely yet is not as dressy as the collar bar or pin and is therefore more appropriate for normal business wear.

COLLAR STYLES

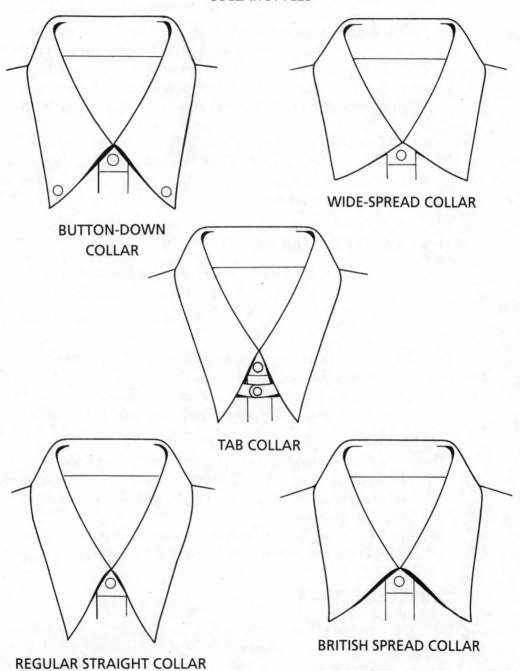

BUTTON-DOWN
COLLAR

WIDE-SPREAD COLLAR

TAB COLLAR

REGULAR STRAIGHT COLLAR

BRITISH SPREAD COLLAR

The Regular Straight Dress Collar: This collar has short, medium or long points and should be considered the core of every man's shirt wardrobe. It looks terrific no matter what the color or pattern. This collar style is correctly worn with virtually any type of jacket regardless of its pattern, fabric or color. Most face shapes and sizes are complimented by its lines.

The British Spread Collar: This collar is considered very dressy and is meant to go with most suit jackets, blazers (especially double-breasted) and sport coats. The wide-spread and slightly curved points which touch at the collar, create its dressy effect.

A SHIRT COLLAR AND TIE GUIDE

The shape of a shirt collar generally determines the tie and tie-knot that should be worn with it. Following are the safest combinations:

- The button-down collar works best with a full or half-Windsor, four-in-hand or a bow tie;
- The straight point collar accommodates half-Windsor or four-in-hand knots and bow tie;
- The tab collar must be worn with the tighter four-in-hand knot;
- The wide-spread collar demands the widest full-Windsor knot;
- The European spread also takes a Windsor knot.

For sartorial history buffs: the term "four-in-hand knot" is said to have originated with the coach drivers in England who rode on the backs of carriages and the Windsor knot, of course, was named after the elegant Duke of Windsor.

Now that we've examined the fundamentals of collars, let's look at some of the ways that they can trip us up and how we can be prepared:

BLOODY COLLAR

Just picture this scene: You have traveled half way across the country to give a major presentation that may affect your next promotion or raise. You arise promptly at 6 A.M. in order to have plenty of time before your

8 A.M. meeting. You shower, shave, and order room service. As you flip up your shirt collar to insert your tie neatly underneath, you fail to notice that the minor nick on your neck has begun to bleed ever so slightly since you removed the piece of tissue that seemed to help stop the bleeding. You now look as though you are a failed suicide attempt. Everyone that you come in contact with will notice—much to the detriment of your presentation and hoped for promotion, raise or sale.

While razors, blades and lathers have improved to nearly eliminate the chance of nicks and cuts, don't forget a time-honored remedy to be packed in your toiletry kit—the styptic pencil. This little lifesaver contains as its active ingredient, aluminum sulfate, and can dry up a cut in seconds. If it's too late for the styptic pencil to come to the rescue, be prepared for emergencies.

Always tuck an extra shirt and tie away in your bag just in case. If the bloodied garment is white, check with the hotel clerk for a drop or two of Wite-Out™ the typewriter correcting fluid, for a cover-up.

COLLAR TOO TIGHT

Even the best dressed and most fastidious of men allow this to happen. Having shirts custom-made may avoid this problem as a good maker will check the collar carefully at the initial fitting.

For any shirt, custom or not, the collar when buttoned should be loose enough to insert one finger between your neck and collar comfortably. If you find you can't do this, have your neck re-measured. You'll likely need a larger collar size.

Aside from slowly strangling yourself, which is bad enough, if your collar is too small, your tie cannot sit properly underneath it, and the points of your shirt will not lay properly.

Attempts to make do with a too-small collar are usually unsuccessful. They include: moving the top button over, enlarging the buttonhole with a razor and even attaching a button to an elasticized ring that fits over the original button. The latter idea is the least offensive, and is better than turning your collar button into a possible lethal projectile every time you cough.

FRAYED COLLAR

Few areas receive as much abuse as the top of your collar at the back of your neck. Unfortunately, it's a case of out-of-sight, out-of-mind. Don't think that if you let your hair grow down over your collar no one will notice. They will. Likewise with turning the collar one-quarter inch. This alternative ends up displaying the tie in back—not acceptable!

So what causes this phenomenon? Several factors. When a shirt is laundered and starched, it is done so flat. Then it's folded over and pressed again—double stress to the fabric. Also, when we put the shirt on we flip up the collar, slip a tie around the neck and fold the collar over this. In addition, the hair on the back of our neck scrapes away at this already weakened area (hair has the tensile strength of aluminum when dry!) from week to week.

So what's the solution? Certainly, you cannot prevent the wear that causes the problem. However, you can make sure to have an adequate supply of shirts to allow for a little relief between wearings.

With some custom-made shirts, you can ask to have the collar replaced for the cost of the fabric and labor—cheaper than a new shirt. A word of warning! No matter what they may tell you—a custom maker CANNOT match the original fabric and color. Therefore, this solution is valid only for adding a new, contrast collar to a colored or patterned shirt body.

The bottom line: Inspect the collar of your shirt before you put it on and toss it in the rag pile if it's starting to give out!

FLY-AWAY COLLAR

When you wear a standard spread collar, the points should rest lightly on your shirt. Two reasons for this not happening are:

- The tie is either too wide or too heavy. When tied, it produces a knot that is too large to fit comfortably under the collar points. Be careful when combining a tie that has been an old friend with a new shirt. Collar point lengths change from time to time, so take this into consideration. If you want to try a different collar style, treat yourself to a new tie for the most coordinated look.

- The collar is missing stays. Stays are the plastic strips that fit inside the thin groove sewn into the underside of a collar point. Most cleaners remove these before pressing to avoid accidentally melting them. They may neglect replacing them and leave you in the lurch if you've packed for a trip without double-checking. Buy plastic replacements (very inexpensive) and always have a couple stowed away in your travel kit.

Brass collar stays also work very well and come in several sizes. Unlike plastic you can't trim them with scissors to fit, but you'll be a lot more careful to remove them when you send your shirts to the laundry.

Two ideas I never thought of were shared with me by a couple of friends: A young clothing maven in North Carolina suggests trying a large paper clip in a pinch and an early mentor of mine at Bloomingdales once told me of a time he was away from home and found that he was missing one of his two collar stays. Ever resourceful, he trimmed the edge of a recently expired credit card to fit. It worked, and he swears he'll still cut his cards in half when they expire but he won't throw the halves away.

CUFFS

There are only three types of shirt cuffs available in the ready-to-wear marketplace:

Barrel Cuff: This is without a doubt the most common style. It is a single-thickness cuff fastened with either one or two buttons. It is always correct, and is easily folded under when a roll-up-your-sleeves look is called for.

French Cuff: This is a long cuff worn folded in half and held together with cuff links. Widely available, this is the dressiest of all the cuff styles. Anyone can wear a French cuff as long as care is taken when selecting the cuff links. The most traditional are made of gold, decorated with a simple design, a small semi-precious stone or monogram. Subtlety is the watchword for cuff links; if you can't lift your arms without help, they are too big!

Convertible Cuff: This is a barrel cuff that has buttonholes on both sides and can be worn with or without cuff links. A bit difficult to find, try a men's specialty store if you require a shirt capable of performing this double duty.

SHIRT FABRICS

There are many types of shirt fabrics: 100% cotton, cotton and polyester blends, silk and all polyester. All cotton and the cotton and polyester blends are the most appropriate for everyday use. The following are the most common and acceptable:

Broadcloth: This is a tightly woven fabric with a simple, plain weave. Both 100% cotton and cotton-blends are used to create this weave. It can be found in a variety of styles, colors and patterns. Generally, it is considered a dressy fabric due to its fine thread, tight weave and slight sheen. "Icy" colors are usually made by adding a drop or two of pigment to this bright white fabric.

Egyptian Cotton: This is considered the finest cotton grown in the world. It is extremely soft and silky to the touch, light and comfortable to wear. Since it absorbs dyes beautifully, it produces colors and subtle patterns second to none. The drawbacks are it is very expensive, wrinkles fairly easily and must be sent to a good laundry for cleaning and pressing. But, having said that, these are fabulous shirts to own and wear, if only for special occasions. Treat yourself to one—you won't regret it.

Oxford Cloth: This is a popular cotton or cotton-blend fabric produced by using two fine crossing yarns with a heavier filling yarn to yield a firm yet soft and very durable finish. It is not considered a dressy fabric and is usually used in button-down collar shirts. It does not pair with formal suit patterns and fabric very well. This fabric can be a real workhorse, holding up to wash after wash; however, only the blends can be cared for at home with relative ease.

Pinpoint Oxford: This is similar to oxford except it is made from much finer yarn and is therefore a more tightly woven fabric resulting in a smoother, silkier, softer and far dressier shirt. It falls comfortably in-between broadcloth and standard oxford cloth in terms of formality. Ask for light starch when having them laundered, and every fourth laundering skip the starch altogether and these shirts will last a lot longer.

Tone on Tone: This is a design woven into fabric using two or more tones of the same color or two or more different patterns in the same color for a subtle, elegant effect. It is used primarily in very dressy shirts. Be careful when considering this fabric because there is no in-between with it: It either looks extremely classy or very cheap. Price and your eye are the only guides.

End-on-End: This is a closely woven fabric with alternating white and colored yarns running both horizontally and vertically. This creates a fine checkered appearance with a flat texture. With a contrasting white collar and/or cuffs, you have a dressy, formal look which is a little different but quite acceptable in business situations.

Sea Island Cotton: This is a fine, lustrous cotton grown mostly in the West Indies as well as on islands off Georgia, South Carolina, Texas and Florida. It is the domestic version of Egyptian cotton with all its fine qualities and features. It also has the added advantage of being grown in the U.S.A.

Cotton Blends: Certain combinations of fibers bring out the best in each. For example, cotton-polyester blend is one most commonly found in stores today. This combination combines the softness of cotton with the easy-care qualities of polyester which makes the choice perfect for a wrinkle-free look when traveling.

Silk: A thread or fabric made from the fine, lustrous fiber produced by the silkworm to form its cocoon. Silk is a strong, resilient fiber and is used to make the finest shirts. Usually too dressy for normal business wear but a fabric that feels and looks luxurious.

 SHIRT FIT

Men buy shirts by neck size and sleeve size since that is how they are sold in virtually all department stores, men's specialty stores or catalogs. Neck sizes vary by one-half-inch increments from 14 to 19 or so, and sleeve sizes range from 30 to 38 in one-inch increases. Exact sizes in sleeve lengths means each size is carried 30, 31, 32, 33 and so forth; average sleeve sizes are not as precise and are given as 32-33, 34-35 and so forth. Exact sizing is usually the best although it demands a larger inventory to be stocked by the seller.

Another element to be considered is body style or cut. The type of cut varies by the manufacturer and even by different lines of the same maker. In general, there are three body styles of shirts available:

- **Fitted:** This style is cut narrower through the chest and body and presents a very trim silhouette.
- **Traditional:** This style is often referred to as a "gentleman's cut," fuller across the chest and not as nipped in at the waist. This cut fits the vast majority of men pretty well.
- **Full:** This style is best exemplified by a Brooks Brothers shirt. These shirts are extremely comfortable, but many men find them a little too roomy, resulting in excess fabric to tuck into their trousers. One co-worker told me he never wears a Brooks Brothers shirt in Chicago, fearing a rogue gust of wind might send him sailing skyward!

✖✖ FINDING THE RIGHT STYLE FOR YOU

If your buttons pull, the placket of your shirt (the double layer of fabric in the front of the shirt through which the buttonholes are cut) doesn't lay flat against your chest or stomach and, thus, horizontal creases may appear. It may not mean you have a weight problem; rather, you may be trying to wear a cut that is not suited to your body type.

On the other hand, if there is too much fabric through the body, a few solutions are available: A tailor can taper a shirt by removing excess fabric from under the armhole down through the shirt's tail. Remember that when we sit down some of us expand, so, when the tailor pins the sides, make sure he allows for this. This alteration is permanent.

As an alternative, darts can be inserted in the back of a shirt to reduce the amount of fabric. The darts are slightly visible but not unsightly and can be removed if necessary. As a general rule, darts work best for removing small amounts of fabric.

BUTTONING UP A BETTER STYLE—NON-DRESS SHIRT WITH A TIE

A flannel shirt with a knit or woven tie is very much at home with a Harris tweed sports coat but it is not considered proper in most business settings.

A fine cotton tartan plaid shirt with a coordinated linen woven or cotton knit tie is super for informal weekend wear, as is the knit polo-type shirt with three-button front placket worn with a properly informal tie.

Denim and chambray shirts are extremely handsome when paired with jeans or khakis. And all sorts of neat, fun ties look great with them. This look is perfect for less dressy business days or weekends.

A WORD ABOUT UNDERSHIRTS

While wearing an undershirt keeps its wearer comfortable and protects expensive outer garments from unsightly perspiration stains, it should be appreciated, but never seen.

Your choice of undershirt styles is limited to crew-neck, V-neck and tank top-singlet. You should try to match the style to the occasion. The crew neck is the best for most business situations. However, when your plans call for you to wear a shirt that is open at the collar, consider switching to a V-neck. This way you get all the benefits without sharing your underwear with the world.

Most military branches and some civilian occupations have uniforms that are open at the neck. Army regulations require a green or olive drab crew-neck T-shirt with open neck fatigues or battle dress uniforms. If you fall into this category, have a few crew-necks for when you "dress up," but try to stick to the vees for day-in-and-day-out use.

Other than its light weight, I have found no major advantage, or proper use, for the tank top unless you work outside and remove your outer shirt regularly.

✖ ✖ ✖

CONTRAST STITCHING

If you own a shirt with contrast stitching, do not wear it with a tie. Never! (This means a shirt where the thread that connects the cuff to the sleeve, pocket to the body, and runs around the collar and down the front placket is of a different color than the body of the garment.) Reserve these shirts for your leisure outfits—perfect for a Texas barbecue, for instance.

 SHORT SLEEVES

In some areas of the country during the summer months, a short-sleeved dress shirt is perfectly acceptable. "Guayaberas," for instance, are beautiful and very practical formal shirts, worn in South America. However, give some North American men a sartorial inch and they will do their very best to take a mile. Just because it's "OK" where you live, don't expect others to automatically accept this form of business dress when you travel. They won't.

This may not make sense but it is one of those "Clothing Enigmas" that serve as an arbitrary rule that you are safer to observe than to ignore.

In most large urban areas the work place is air conditioned, as are most cars and homes. There simply is no real reason to wear short sleeves. If the heat bothers you, try a cotton or good cotton-blend shirt with long sleeves. You'll be surprised at how comfortable they can be.

If you need to keep the wrist area clear of fabric for work-related reasons, fold the cuff of your long- sleeved shirt under into the sleeve; don't roll it up on the outside. Folding it under will keep it up and still present a neat appearance.

 IF YOU ARE BOARDROOM BOUND

If you are working your way into the boardroom, avoid:

- aviator shirts with epaulets (unless, of course, you are a pilot);
- front pockets with flaps and buttons;
- any type of contrasting stitching or trim;

• a pattern that falls outside of the generally accepted stripes, tatter-sall, plaids, pinstripes, pencil stripes, university stripes or—for the more adventurous—a bold stripe body with white collar and cuffs.

✖ ✖ ✖

On clean-shirt day
he went abroad,
and paid visits.

—Samuel Johnson
Boswell's *Life of Dr. Johnson*

Special Order, Made-to-Measure, and Custom—Just for You

The most expensive and the most precise way to achieve the look and fit that is right for you is to have it made.

Far too many myths and altogether too much misinformation have surrounded the idea of having a suit, sport coat or shirt made especially for you. Visions of the Great Gadsby, an oil baron, European Lord or other positioned person still permeate the notion of "custom."

If you answer yes to any of the following questions, then you should seriously consider one of the several options available as an alternative to ready to wear: Special Order, Made-to-Measure and Custom. Let's begin with the qualifying questions:

- Do you have difficulty finding your size in most retail stores?
- Would you like to see a greater selection of colors or patterns?
- Are you too busy to shop around?
- Do you have a physical feature that makes fitting difficult?
- Does a unique styling feature appeal to you?
- Do you enjoy personal attention?
- Can you afford to pay a little more for exactly what you want?
- Do you want the best possible in all things?
- Does your build require special attention to fit correctly?

An answer of yes suggests that you would enjoy learning about the world of clothing that is not made for the average person in terms of size, taste, fit, construction or even price. To begin with, we must clearly understand that there is a difference between the terms Special Order, Made-To-Measure, and Custom.

SPECIAL ORDER

Whether we are talking about shirts or suits/sports coats, most good men's specialty stores and exceptionally good men's departments in larger specialty/department stores can order garments for you that do not exist in their normal inventory. The choices that you will be offered will allow you to create an article of clothing uniquely yours that fits the way you want it to.

In a shirt the choices will probably be limited to the following: six to eight collar styles, three or four body models, two or three cuff types as well as monogram and shirt pocket options for you to choose from. All of which will be available in a very wide variety of fabrics and colors. And, of course, in whatever collar and sleeve length combination you might need to ensure a correct fit.

A special order suit will allow you to decide not only what size jacket and pant waist is perfect for you, as opposed to the standard drop normally available on the rack, but, also, silhouette (with limited alterations to the standard pattern); lining type (full or half or fancy); choice of vent (center, side or closed); pant model (plain front, forward or reverse pleats); pant linings (crotch, half lined to the knee or fully lined) and vested or two piece model. As long as your size is fairly regular, (i.e. jacket and pant are a size for which a pattern already exists in the manufacturer's files) special order is "tailor made" for you . Amazingly, the cost is not much more than if you bought the suit or shirt off of the store's shelf or suit rack. The delivery time is four to six weeks depending on the maker selected.

MADE-TO-MEASURE

The fabrics, patterns and colors from which to choose are every bit as bountiful as special order but the range of options increases to include pocket treatments either inside or outside the jacket and lowering or raising of the trouser waistband. The biggest difference between the two is in the number of measurements taken which, therefore, results in a better fit. In addition to the jacket chest size and pant waist, the following measurements will be taken as well:

- **Jacket:** chest, over-arm, waist, seat, full length, back, point-to-point, sleeve length and half-waist as well as adjustments for a high or a low shoulder and whether to raise, lower or shorten the collar.

- **Trouser:** rise, outseam, inseam, waist, abdomen, seat, knee, bottom and, if necessary, adjustments for bow legs and a high or low hip.

The cost is ten to twenty percent higher than off the rack and the time needed for delivery is from six to twelve weeks. Since a pattern in being created for you, the first order takes the longest time to fulfill; after that, only small changes due to fine tuning or weight fluctuations are necessary.

CUSTOM

True custom or "Bespoke" clothing does all of the above and then some. If ritual and absolute precision are for you, and time and money are no object, *then this is the experience of a lifetime.*

Shirt: A custom shirt as a rule will include at least 12 measurements: 1. weight; 2. shoulder line; 3. chest; 4. waist; 5. hips; 6. arms; 7. wrists; 8. neck; 9. collar front height; 10. collar back height; 11. shirt length overall; 12. your height.

- The swatch selection increases dramatically from a few to literally hundreds.
- The option to specify vertical stripes, to edge stitch the collar and to create a box or sleeve pleat are offered.
- On average, eleven collar styles, six pocket styles and six cuff styles are available. With all these variables, a shirt takes approximately three to six weeks from ordering to delivery.
- One extremely attractive option, currently available, is the ability to have one shirt of your order completed in only about a week, changes can be made and then the balance of the order comes in a short time later just the way you want them. This is a wonderful way to have shirts made.

Suit: A custom suit takes into consideration all of the measurements needed for a special order and made-to measure suit, plus many more. Overall as many as a score or more, including shoulder angle; arm pitch;

posture; blades in or out; and coat length; this is just a partial listing of a suit guaranteed to follow every contour and nuance of your body.

You should be in no rush for the garment; count on an average of two months for the whole process to be complete from first fitting to final delivery. Normally three visits to the tailor are required:

- The first for the detailed measurements and to choose between the many bolts or fabric swatches available (if they cannot verify availability on the spot, select a strong second choice in the event the manufacturer has run out of a particular fabric; until the fabric is reserved, you are not sure of getting your first choice; get a price quote to include any extras you may have chosen to add; be sure to write down the number of the fabric you have selected to double check when the garment arrives months later).

- The second to adjust the unfinished garment (often you will be trying on a sleeveless, white cotton muslin prototype) or the actual garment without sleeves in order to make adjustments and to set the sleeves to the pitch (the forward or rearward positioning) of your arms.

- And the final session, at last recognizable as a suit, is the time for a final check. Even though you may feel like old friends, try everything on and check for all the options you requested. If all has gone well, this attention will have produced a garment of unequaled quality and comfort that is yours alone.

Andy Manwani, a wardrobe consultant, has helped thousands of men design a personal look during his more than two decades of working in the men's clothing field. I think he sums up what has been said rather nicely: "If you want the best fit, a selection of luxurious fabrics, a variety of patterns and unlimited style choices, you can create an individual statement of who you are by taking advantage of custom or made-to-measure clothing. Ready to wear cannot compare."

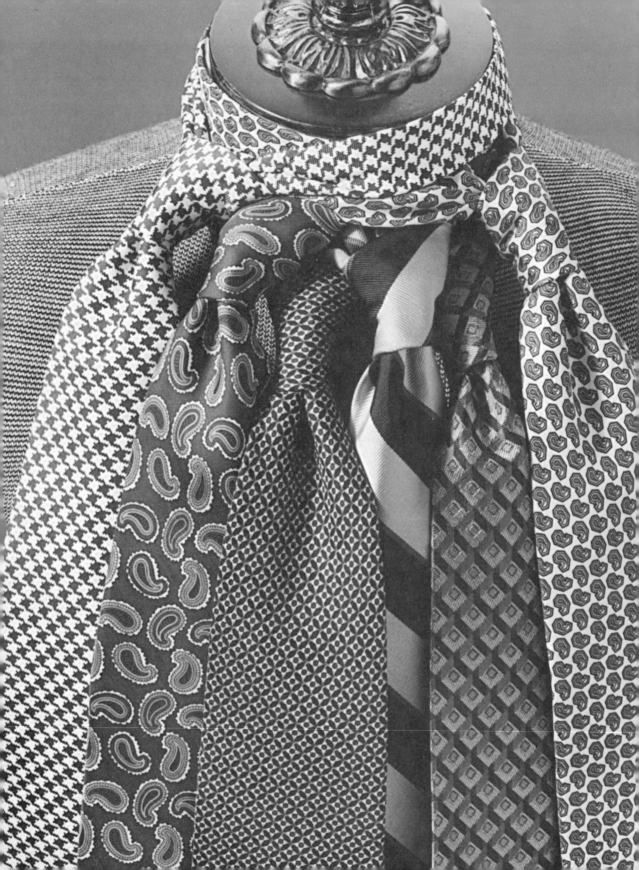

6 | The Ties Have It

Axiom: There's no such thing as a "well, it's okay" tie. Ties either work for you or they work against you—with a vengeance!

It's also a fact that many men delegate the chore of picking their ties to the women in their lives: wives, lovers and secretaries. Mothers and sisters also contribute their fair share to a man's tie rack. Now a number of men will shrug, "But women have an eye for these things. They're more 'sensitive' to color." There may be some truth to this. But the logic is debatable and to exercise it constantly is to rob yourself of the skills you need to master your own selection of this extremely important item of apparel. No pain, no gain; use it or lose it. It's up to you. A woman in your life can without doubt add an invaluable opinion but you shouldn't be passing the buck when it comes to an item that is considered "you."

If you're one of the great number of men who are accustomed to leaving their apparel selections to the women in their lives, it may be a good idea to shop with them and ask what it is they like about one necktie as opposed to another. With just a little work you can be the best at making selections that constitute perfect taste and—equally important—picking the neckwear that subtly expresses what is special about the inner you.

In this chapter, you will learn the insider's tips of the trade; use them to create your own personal style. But first, let's start at the beginning, literally, with the origin of neckties.

 A SHORT HISTORY LESSON

When they visited Paris in the mid-1600's, a regiment of superstitious Croats (from what is now Croatia) wore silk kerchiefs as talismans to ward off blows to the throat. Louie XIV admired the brightly colored silk worn by the mercenaries and soon produced one of his own. Embroidered and tied with a simple knot, this new style was named the "cravat" (the French word for Croat). The nobility of neckwear quickly caught on, and the tying of the tie became an entire regimen in and of itself. By the 18th Century, the cravat had evolved into the slender rectangle with a diamond-shaped tip that we associate with neckwear today. The ready-made tie began competing with the handmade cravat and eventually took over the neckwear market.

A WALKING TOUR OF THE NECKTIE

The first thing to do to tame this monster known as the necktie is to walk around it and get to know its parts, what makes it work, what makes it cheap or expensive and so forth:

Length: The average tie is between 54" and 56" in length. If a man is very tall (6'3" or over), has a very large neck or is built so that most of his height is in his torso, this length may not be enough. Longer ties are available for the man who needs a bit more. These ties are 60" long and come in a wide range of colors and patterns.

Width: At present, about four inches of tie width is fashionable. Don't expect it to change all that much any time soon. I think it will remain at between three-and-one-half to, at most, four-and-one-fourth inches unless some major unforeseen change takes place in the men's clothing industry. The most important consideration is the proportion of the necktie and the lapel width. As an easy-to-follow and remember rule of thumb, hold the widest part of your tie up against the lapel of the jacket with which you plan to wear it. They should match almost exactly. This only works with a single-breasted, notched lapel; don't try it with a peaked lapel—it won't work.

Fabric: Choose natural fibers such as silk, wool and cotton. Because natural fibers absorb dyes so well, they tend to create very beautiful colorations with very subtle nuances occurring in the printing, weaving or screening process. Since many of the wool ties are best in winter and fall and cotton should be kept exclusively for summertime wear, the overwhelming choice for ties is silk for year-round wear. Silk knots well, com-

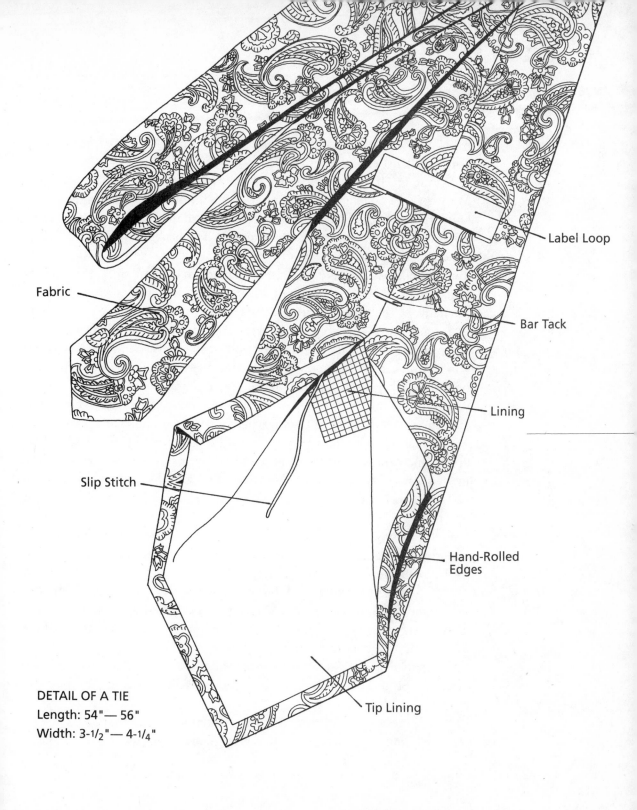

Label Loop

Fabric

Bar Tack

Lining

Slip Stitch

Hand-Rolled
Edges

Tip Lining

DETAIL OF A TIE
Length: 54" — 56"
Width: 3-1/2" — 4-1/4"

presses upon itself to form a compact tasteful little bud that fits perfectly under the shirt collar points.

Lining: The tie's lining adds the body and heft that make a good knot. Many people erroneously assume that the number of gold stripes on the lining indicates the quality of the tie. In fact, the stripes are simply a measure of how heavy that particular lining is. The heavier the silk, the lighter the coarse wool lining.

Label Loop: Unlike the label on the back of your shirt, this label is functional and not just a form of advertising. While it does routinely carry the name of the manufacturer or the retailer, or both, its true value lies in its intended use—to hold the narrow end of the necktie neatly in place when tied. Simply slide the narrow end of the tie through the label after you've finished tying the knot and it will stay neat and out of sight without any further attention. If you are very tall and the loop is too low for you to insert the narrow end after tying the knot, it is a relatively minor alteration to have it moved up to where it can be useful.

Bar Tack: Handmade ties should be bar tacked to maintain their appearance and symmetrical shape. Look for a smallish—about one-half inch or less—stitch anchoring the seam running the length of the tie at both ends. This keeps the tie from coming undone after many months of wear and tear.

Tip Lining: Most ties have a lightweight silk lining in both ends; this is a finishing touch that is purely cosmetic. Some ties of heavy silk (such as the exquisite 7-Folds) are not lined to the tip.

Slip Stitch: A long thread that runs the length of the tie on the underside of the tie joining the fabric. Made up of individual stitches, they will be uneven and fairly loose. The end of this stitch can be found at the end of the tie by turning it over and looking for the knotted end.

Hand-Rolled Edges: A tie that is rolled and hemmed by hand has a better shape and maintains it longer. This is seen at either end of the tie at the tip.

Lifelines: Loops of thread at the ends of some ties that allow the tie to stretch and "give" when knotted after many wearings.

✖ ✖ ✖

Solid

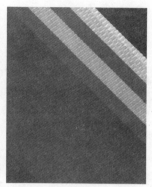
Repp Stripe

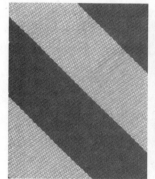
Regimental Stripe

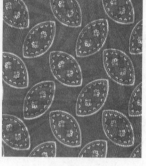
Foulard

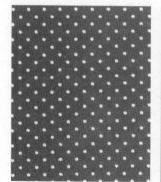
Dots

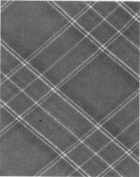
Plaid

MAJOR NECKTIE PATTERNS AND THEIR APPROPRIATENESS

Solid: A single color in silk, wool, cotton or a blend of fibers. A deep, rich burgundy is a "must have" for all men. *Simple, yet elegant.*

Repp Stripe: Any tie with diagonal stripes made of a cross-weave fabric. *Business wear.*

Regimental Stripe: Once different than the repp, it is now practically the same thing. Originally it was a striped tie carrying the colors of a British gentleman's old army regiment or school. In England, it is poor form to wear the stripes of a regiment in which you did not serve. *Business wear.*

Foulard: A lightweight silk in twill weave. It is usually made up of small, regularly spaced designs such as circles, ovals, diamonds or a combination of shapes on a solid background. *Business wear/Dressy.*

Dots: Ranging downward in size from approximately the diameter of a dime to mini- and micro-dots; the smaller the dot, the dressier the look. *Dressy.*

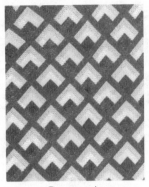

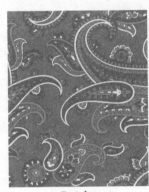

Geometric   *Paisley*

Plaid: Usually of wool for winter wear or cotton for summer, it is a box-like design formed of stripes running vertically and horizontally and often associated with a particular Scottish tartan. *Casual.*

Geometric: This can be everything from an enlarged diamond pattern to a crisscross or vertically striped pattern. *Casual.*

Paisley: Adopted from colorful and intricate Kashmir shawls, the first commercial printing took place in Paisley, Scotland. Paisley can look very sporty if the colors are bright to very elegant if the colors are subdued. Because of the combination of colors, this pattern can go with a variety of looks. *Casual/Elegant.*

Conversational: Any design that represents an item or activity showing affiliation or affection. Nichol Miller's occupation and leisure time motifs; a tie covered with elegantly printed string instruments worn by a concert violinist; a National Wildlife Federation tie with beautifully screened loons are all examples of this very popular style. *Casual.*

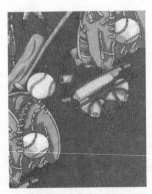

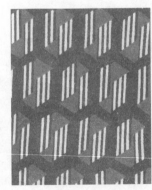

Conversational   *Retro Looks*

Retro Looks: Exaggerated, oversized patterns reminiscent of the styles popular during the thirties and forties. Hand painted hula dancers or bright, giant shapes allow for a lot of self-expression. *Casual.*

Knit: Made of silk or wool with a distinctly woven appearance. Yellow or burgundy silk pairs up

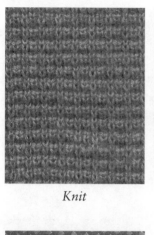
Knit

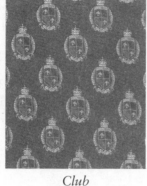
Club

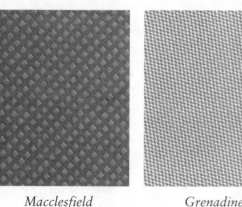

Macclesfield

Grenadine

nicely with a navy business suit for a great look. A knit wool tie is almost always better worn with a sports coat. *Dressy/Casual.*

Club: Most often made of silk, it has a dark background upon which woven patterns of heraldic devices or sporting symbols are diagonally repeated. Originally British and associated with men's clubs, it is now a way of expressing any association with an organization, cause or activity. *Casual.*

Macclesfield: An open-weave silk, usually in contrasting tones such as gray and black. *Elegant.*

Grenadine: A thin, loosely woven, lightweight silk with a pronounced irregular surface. *Dressy.*

COMBINING COATS, TIES AND SHIRTS
MIXING PATTERNS

Gone are the days of plain and boring. Today, men are combining two and even three patterns with sophisticated effectiveness. There are exceptions to every rule, so here are some guidelines to follow as you create the look that is yours alone, the look that expresses who you are or how you want others to see you:

Combine Compatible Fabrics: Fabrics vary in texture, finish and weight and all pieces should be consistent. For example, a worsted wool suit with a cotton broadcloth shirt and a fine silk tie. Or, a herringbone tweed sport coat with an oxford cloth button-down and a woven or knit wool tie.

Contrast: It always looks best to have some contrast between the suit and shirt, and the shirt and tie. Lack of contrast can result in an overall monochromatic effect that is too dull and uninteresting.

CHART FOR COMBINING

SUIT	SHIRT	TIE
To Create Contrast:		
Dark	Light	Bright Medium-Dark
Medium	Light	Dark
Light	Medium	Dark
To Combine Three Solids:		
Solid	Solid	Solid
To Combine Two Solids and One Pattern:		
Solid	Solid	Pattern
Solid	Pattern	Solid
Pattern	Solid	Solid
To Combine Two Patterns and One Solid:		
Solid	Pattern	Pattern
Pattern	Solid	Pattern
Pattern	Pattern	Solid
To Combine Three Patterns:		
Pinstripe	Average Stripe	Foulard
Glen Plaid	Bold Stripe	Club
Herringbone	Two Color Stripe	Paisley

Some Words of Caution When Combining More Than Two Patterns

- If more than one pattern is used, care should be taken to provide contrast in the scale, such as small versus large.
- Colors must blend. One color must be repeated in all three patterns. For example, a suit, shirt and tie all have a complimentary shade of blue in them.
- Two stripes must be of different widths, such as wide versus narrow.
- Avoid a combination so perfect that it becomes a uniform always worn the same way and noticed.

MAJOR NECKTIE KNOT STYLES

There are only three distinctly different ways to tie a necktie, and most men only know one—the one they learned when they were first forced to wear a tie. Because of a number of factors—change in physique, new styles of shirt collars or just appropriateness—learning a different knot tying technique makes sense. (See pages 176-177.) The three major knot styles are:

✖✖ WINDSOR

This knot fills the space between wide-spread collar points, and it takes a lot of fabric to make it. If your ties hang too low, this knot can help, but it will not fit under the newer shirt collar styles and is too large for small or thin face shapes.

How to tie:

1. Begin with the wide end of the tie a little more than a foot longer on the right side...
2. Cross wide end over and back underneath narrow end...
3. Bring up and turn down through loop...
4. Repeat, bringing wide end up and back through loop on other side of knot...
5. Pass wide end around front...

✖✖
✖✖

6. Then up through the loop…

7. Finally, down through the knot in front. Tighten carefully by sliding up the knot until it is drawn up tight beneath the collar.

✖✖ **HALF-WINDSOR**

This knot is more appropriate for standard spread collars, either straight or button-down. It should also be used with lighter weight silk ties to add bulk to the look of the tie. Identified by its triangular shape and symmetrical look, it looks good on most men.

How to tie:

1. Begin with wide end of tie on your right and extending about a foot below the narrow end…

2. Cross wide end over the narrow end and turn back underneath…

3. Bring up and then down through loop…

4. Pass wide end around front from left to right…

5. Then, up through loop…

6. And down through knot in front. Tighten carefully and draw up to collar.

✖✖ **FOUR-IN-HAND**

This knot is especially good for tall men who need the extra length, for men with round face shapes, for use with heavyweight fabrics, and for small spread collars like the long point, tab or pinned collar.

How to tie:

1. Start with the wide end of the tie on your right and extending a little less than a foot below the narrow end…

2. Cross wide end over narrow end and back underneath…

3. Continue around, passing wide end across front of narrow once more…

4. Pass wide end up through loop…

5. Holding front of knot loose with index finger, pass wide end down through loop in front…

6. Remove finger and tighten knot carefully. Draw up tight to collar by holding narrow end and sliding knot up snugly.

TWO ALTERNATIVES TO THE NECKTIE
BOW TIE

People who wish to wear bow ties as part of their business persona generally know how to tie them; most men only wear a bow tie as part of a formal ensemble. For those who have struggled to tie their bow tie 15 minutes before leaving for a black tie affair, here is a little help. To put you in the correct frame of mind, remember it is exactly the same motion as tying your shoe.

How to tie:

1. Start with end in left hand extending one and one-half inches below that in your right hand…
2. Cross longer end over shorter and pass up through loop. Basically tie an overhand knot…
3. Form front loop of bow by doubling up shorter, hanging end and placing across collar points…
4. Hold this loop with thumb and forefinger of left hand. Drop long end down over front…
5. Place right forefinger, pointing up, on bottom half of hanging part. Pass up behind front loop and…
6. Poke resulting loop through knot behind front loop (see illustration). Even the ends by pulling gently on flat ends and tighten by pulling on the looped ends until you're satisfied.

ASCOT

This is a wonderful, elegant and comfortable alternative to wear when the situation calls for being dressed up but your normal work uniform simply won't do, such as an office Christmas party, major horse racing event or informal garden wedding.

How to tie:

1. Start with the right end extending six inches below the left end...
2. Cross the right end over the left and back underneath...
3. Continue around, passing right end across front of left end once more...
4. Pass right end up through loop at neck...
5. Bring right end down and over left end...
6. Adjust bib at throat to cover the knot. Tuck ascot points under shirt front leaving top two buttons open.

COMBINING COAT AND TIE

Everyone uses pretty much the same procedure when selecting a necktie to go with a jacket, regardless of whether it is a suit jacket or sports coat. But, as far as we know, no one has ever attempted to put it down in a step-by-step formula. Following, then, is a universal method that any man can use to create his own stylish look.

For the purpose of our understanding, let's assume we are looking at a navy blue suit with very subtle burgundy and teal (a combination of blue and green) stripes running throughout; the stripes are separated by a faint white beaded pinstripe. Our shirt is solid white.

The four steps are:

1. Identify. To begin with, you must learn to look at the jacket for which you are choosing a necktie. Not just see it, but closely *Look At It.* If that means finding a location in the store with better than average lighting, do it. Every jacket has a base color—the one you would say it is from three feet away. Up close, though, look carefully and you may be surprised to see all sorts of other colors in the fabric: accent stripes, box-like windowpane plaids, color nubs and slubs or flecks of color woven throughout. If color blindness limits your color identification, don't be afraid to ask for help. Other shoppers, male or female, store clerks or friends and family will be more than happy to assist. Once you know what various colors are present and you are consciously aware of them, you are ready to move on to the next step. Remember in our example, the colors are navy blue (the background), white (the beaded pinstripe) and burgundy and teal (the subtle stripes).

   2. Isolate. Decide which of the colors you want to "pull out" or accent. Using our example, we decide to select the burgundy. At this point, you must determine the chosen color's exact shading; many colors have ranges of brightness and subtlety, warmth and coolness. Our burgundy is a very traditional shade, resembling the color of a very good wine. This now becomes the color of our search.

   3. Amplify. To amplify we must simply find more of it, and the easiest way is to find that color in a necktie—either in the background color or in the design of the tie. Don't look for an absolutely perfect match; it won't matter too much because your eye does something called color compensation when scanning from a jacket across another field of color like a shirt and then onto a third field of color with a tie. Your eyes compensate for the color differences and see harmony. This is the time to wander around looking at the seemingly endless display of neckties on tables, hanging spinners, and in cases (one of my favorite stores has approximately

---

A FINE POINT OF TIE TYING: CREATING THE DIMPLE

   A dimple is a small indentation or crease in the middle of the tie, found just beneath the knot itself. This crease allows the tie to take on a certain elegant drape with just the right amount of fullness and causes the tie to jut out exuding confidence.

   To get a dimple, make sure that you have tied the tie without twisting either side of it in the process. Next, insert your index finger under the knot, centered between the edges of the wide end of the tie; at the same time, gently compress the edges of the tie as you pull it through, thus creating a crease. As you tighten the tie, gradually slip your finger out. A perfect dimple will remain.

9,000 ties on display at any one time). By knowing exactly what color you are looking for the choices are easily whittled down to a manageable number (you easily eliminate, for example, a medium blue tie with a dia-mond-shaped pattern containing orange and yellow). We have found a match for our example—a true burgundy tie with a slight bit of texture containing a foulard pattern which is blue and white concentric circles.

4. Coordinate and Accent. Now is the time to take the candidates over to the jacket. Insert the shirt into the opening in the jacket so it looks like you are wearing it. Then, take each tie, twisting and pinching it so that it fits under the shirt collar points, and see how you react to it. If you like it, move it to the right as a possibility and try the next one. If you don't like it, put it off to the left and start a reject pile. Go through and see how you've done. If they all look fine, then begin to fine tune as to design size and shape, to fit your personality and the mood to be created. If you don't like any, look at what you selected and see where you went wrong. Choose and bring back another group and try step four again. Remember the white shirt we are using as a backdrop; if it is not working as well with the jacket as we would have liked, it may be time to look at blue, ecru, pink or a stripe on a white, off-white or pastel background.

This is a very simplified approach to combining. Here are a few refinements to the basic formula to help fine tune your eye and to expand your thinking on the subject:

- Suit and shirt should contrast; the necktie "ties" the two colors together.
- Ties in red, burgundy, navy, teal and yellow provide a compatible accent to most suit colors.
- A solid suit allows for more flexibility when combining a patterned shirt and tie.
- Never underestimate the power of a crisp, pure white shirt with almost any tie that contains a drop of white in the pattern.
- Two patterns will work together if one is close or fine and the other is open or broad. An open shirt pattern allows the tighter tie pattern to dominate for a workable combination.

- Boldly colored shirt stripes require more background color in the tie or a paisley to balance the boldness.
- A necktie that picks up the major colors of the suit and shirt will create an eye-catching focal point.

INSIDER'S TIPS OF THE TRADE

You should be well on your way now to mastering the tie, so let's take a look at some of those insider's tips that we mentioned earlier.

Three or More Patterns in One Tie

Often, a misguided attempt to produce a necktie that will appeal to everyone. Usually it ends up a tie that appeals to no one.

Tie Tying Troubles

There are three ways to botch it in this very visible area of dressing:

- First is the tie's fabrication. If the tie has a lot of polyester in it, it has a heavier lining to keep its shape. Hence, a very out-of-proportion knot results.

- Second, the Windsor knot (as described earlier, a large knot popularized by the late Duke of Windsor) is very formal, symmetrical and extremely stylish when worn with a spread collar. It should not be worn with button-down collars or a collar bar, pin or tab collar.

- Third, if the ends of your tie are nearly even before you begin the knot, odds are that when you finish the knot it will not be the proper length. If you are of average height, the wide end of your tie should be approximately nine and one-half to ten and one-half inches longer when first draped around your neck before you begin to tie it.

Tie Too Short

Your tie must come down to your belt line! Your tie MUST come down to your belt line. This is not arbitrary, this is not negotiable—your tie must come down to your belt line. Hollywood wardrobers have known for years that if you want to make a man look like a rube who has fallen off a turnip truck on his first trip to town, all they have to do is shorten his tie by three inches and let his stomach hang out. It works every time. Next time you watch a movie and see a character not quite up to snuff, look closely and you will see that they may have done this to present him that way.

The only leeway that is allowed as to the length of the tie is the width of the belt. As long as the tip of the tie is between the upper and lower edges of the belt, you're still okay. If you choose to wear braces/suspenders instead of a belt, then you don't have the aforementioned safety zone, so make sure you reach down to the top of the trouser's waistband. If you go a bit longer, that is all right, too. How long is too long? If the end of your tie interferes with the orderly operation of your zipper, then it's too long.

The Long and Short of It

Most ties are made to measure 56-1/2 inches when laid out end-to-end. If you happen to be the exact height and weight the tie manufacturers had in mind, your tie would end just at the top of your belt buckle or ever so slightly below the top. When tied, the narrow end should still fit through the loop on the back of your tie to help keep it in place. If not, a qualified tailor can move the loop for you. If your tie is still too short, you should investigate the big and tall men's shops for ties specially designed for the bigger guy.

Tie Too Wide or Too Narrow

Pierre Cardin was quoted as saying, "In men's fashion, the look changes every five years. But on the streets, it changes every ten years." Don't take this designer's very astute observation and distort it to mean that you can put a tie in the back of your closet, pull it out a decade later, wear it and assume no one will know it's ten years old. They will know it's old; don't do it!

Tie widths correspond very closely to the width of a man's suit or sport coat lapels. To tell if a tie is appropriate with a particular jacket, hold the wide end of your tie up against the widest part of the jacket's lapel. The tie should not be wider than the lapel. It can be a bit narrower, but not too much.

If you have a prized possession that you don't want to part with, take advantage of the cost-effective services of a qualified tailor who will recut your old pal to today's standards of around three and one-half inches. If you are unable to find someone in your area, a company that can help is:

Tiecrafters, Inc.
252 West 29th Street
New York, NY 10001

TIE TACKS

A tie tack is just what the names implies. It has a pointed end that you push through the center of both ends of your necktie. Though the everyday variety has a flat or rounded head, most tie tacks are fancier. Many are embellished with monograms, diamonds or pearls. In order to accomplish its mission—namely to hold the tie in place—the pointed end has to be pushed into something and, fortunately, the inventors did not choose your chest. Instead, it fits into a small metal clip that is connected by a fine chain to a bar that fits into your button hole.

Men seem to either wear tie tacks frequently—and if that's their personal statement, that's okay—or they almost never wear one. Owning a tie tack, though, can be something of a self-fulfilling prophecy. Once you have decided to wear it, you must always wear it as it puts a hole in the center of your tie. It does limit your dressing options which is not usually an advantage, especially with a fine silk tie that costs $35 to $120. Poking a hole in its most visible part is a shame!

✖ ✖ ✖

BOW TIES: CAN THEY BE WORN FOR BUSINESS?

The answer is a qualified yes. You will find very successful men who prefer the bow tie over the more conventional cravat in just about every profession. But because it's a very visible form of expression, be sure that it is in keeping with the image you wish to convey. If you are in a somewhat creative field, the bow tie will convey an air of uniqueness. An academic will send out the message "I am an independent thinker." For much more practical reasons, doctors who choose to wear a bow tie claim it doesn't get in their way when examining a patient. Just be aware of the circumstances and act accordingly.

✖ ✖ ✖

"Men who have learned how to mix patterns
have mastered something very important.
A tie is one of the best forms of
self-expression a man has…"

—Bill Blass

Exceptionally Good Shirt and Tie Combos

✖ ✖ ✖

There is a great deal of trial and error in learning to combine shirts and ties especially when they both have a significant pattern. Trying to tell you how it is done or what is right or wrong without the actual pieces in hand to visualize is as difficult as trying to herd cats into another room. The nuances, differences in size or proportion and color subtleties are enormous to say the least. What is bold to one may be pale to another; what I consider small-medium may seem too large to you.

If you are serious about trying your own hand at creating a style that is uniquely yours, then I applaud you and will do all I can to help you do just that. For comfort, begin with things you already own but rarely wear because you don't seem to have anything that goes with it; reading through the following suggestions may give you an idea or two with which to experiment. Just lay the shirt flat in a well-lit area, spread out all of your ties and try some of the following (remember, you are not supposed to like every possible, technically-correct combination; it should go together in a way that is pleasing to your eye).

SHIRTS

1. moderate to bold stripes widely spaced team with

2. any pin-striped, subtle pattern shirt looks great with

TIE IDEAS TO GET YOU GOING

a tie with more background color than pattern

a deep-toned tie with wide stripes or neat-foulard pattern. Or try an unusual abstract or hand-painted

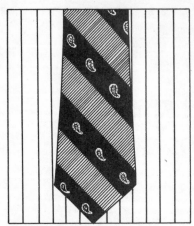

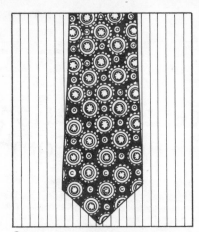

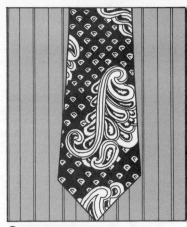

1 Shirt: Moderate to bold stripes
Tie: More background color than pattern

2 Shirt: Pin striped, subtle pattern
Tie: Deep toned with wide stripes or neat-foulard pattern

3 Shirt: Colored with thin widely-spaced accent color stripe
Tie: Bright, bold paisley or all-over pattern to pick up accents

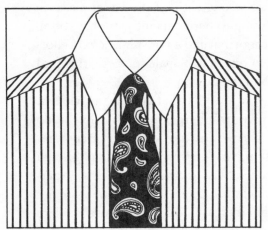

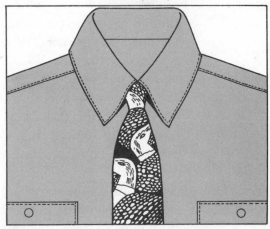

4 Shirt: Bold or thick stripe with contrast white color
Tie: Bold all-over pattern such as paisley or spaced foulard

5 Shirt: Fun denim or chambray work shirt
Tie: Conversational with message or light-hearted tone

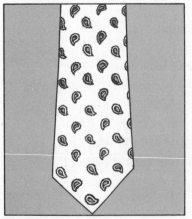

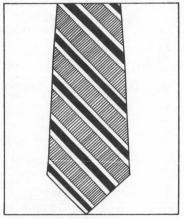

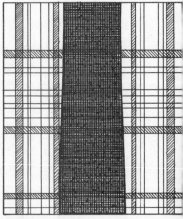

6 Shirt: Chambray or sherbet colored
Tie: Light colored; picks up shirt color in its pattern

7 Shirt: Solid white
Tie: Dash of white in pattern

8 Shirt: Bold plaid
Tie: Complimentary colored, medium toned, knit solid

SHIRTS

**TIE IDEAS
TO GET YOU GOING**

3. a colored shirt with thin, widely spaced accent color stripes needs

a bright, bold paisley tie or other all-over pattern which picks up the colors in the stripes

4. bold or thick striped shirts with a contrasting white collar pair well with

a bold all over pattern such as a paisley or a widely spaced patterned tie

5. a fun denim or heavy chambray work shirt looks great well with

a conversational tie with a message or a light hearted tone. For a real change try a western string tie

6. a chambray or sherbet colored shirt is fantastic with

a light colored tie that picks up the shirt color in its pattern or a compatible bold-bar stripe

7. a solid white shirt

is a "No Brainer," virtually anything goes. A dash of white in the pattern really sets off the combination. Vary the pattern to create dressy or casual effects.

8. a bold, plaid shirt can be worn with

a complimentary colored, medium-toned, knit solid or textured club tie

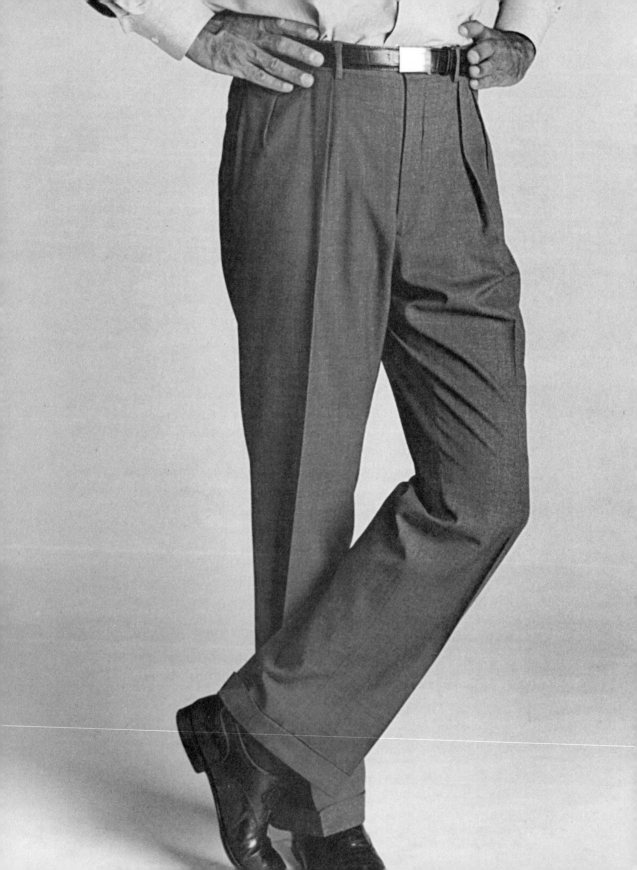

7 | One Leg at a Time: Trousers— Cuts and Cuffs

Few items of apparel are more critical to the way a man feels—and looks—than his trousers. Everything else may be perfect, but if your waistband is compressing you like a Victorian bone corset, if your thighs are numb from loss of circulation, if you're hiking them up or pulling them down, if the seam on your seat is threatening to split open, it's definitely time for a change.

If you should doubt the importance of trousers, remember that we grow in and out of them faster than anything else we wear. The constant battle against the forces of gravity can never be won completely, and so hardly a year passes when we are not reminded by Mother Nature that it's, alas, time for another adjustment. Though the fitness fans among us aren't confronted as often, they, too, must eventually deal with expanding tape measurements.

You need the right trousers for the right look. Actually, the best fit is probably one that lets you forget about your trousers entirely. Easy is the operative word. After all, you've got enough to worry about in your busy, competitive life without having to "sweat it"—literally!

When it comes to pants, the facts really aren't too tough to tackle. A few simple rules will get you by comfortably for the rest of your life.

Before we go over these rules, though, let's examine trouser fabrics for both dress and casual wear and then take a look at pleats.

TROUSER FABRICS

When people talk about fabrics, the feature they most often refer to is the finish. How the garment feels is determined by its finish. There are four major finishes:

✖✖
✖✖

1. **Clear Finish:** When a person says they cannot wear wool because it itches, the finish they want is a clear finish. It is smooth to the touch and free of projecting fiber or fuzziness.
2. **Mill Finish:** Here, the fabric is still soft, but slightly napped.
3. **Semi-Milled Finish:** This fabric is between a clear and a milled finish in feeling with a slight amount of napping to the touch
4. **Flannel Finish:** This fabric is still very soft to the touch but, because of an obvious napped surface, it is "hairier" than the others and can cause discomfort when worn next to the skin of sensitive people.

✖✖   THE MOST COMMON WEAVES AND FABRICS USED TO MAKE MEN'S TROUSERS

DRESS

Worsted: The worsted system of spinning uses long, uniform length fibers that are combed to lie parallel and are tightly twisted together. They are long-wearing, smooth and can be made into very lightweight trousers. This is the term to use when referring to goods that are not itchy and have no nap.

Gabardine: A durable, firmly woven, twill worsted fabric with a clear, hard finish showing single diagonal lines running from bottom left to top right on the face of the fabric. It holds a crease very well and can be comfortably worn ten months of the year.

Flannel: A slightly heavier, soft, luxurious fabric with a napped finish.

Hopsacking: A coarse, open basket weave cloth made primarily of wool.

Cavalry Twill: A strong, rugged cloth made with a pronounced raised cord with a diagonal twill running from lower left to upper right at between a 45 to 63 degree angle. Originally worn in the early 1900s for riding breeches.

Tropical Weight Wool: A lightweight worsted fabric woven from fine yarns primarily in plain weaves. These clear finished fabrics are ideal for warm weather clothing.

Faille Cloth: A slightly ribbed, woven fabric of silk, cotton or rayon.

Wool/Blends: The yarn obtained from the combination of two or more different fibers, natural or man-made. A blend of wool and polyester is often selected for its wrinkle resistance.

CASUAL

Corduroy: A cotton fabric with narrow or wide wales with a velvety surface.

Denim: Strong, washable cotton fabric in a twill weave. It was first made in the French town of Nimes ("de Nimes" meaning from Nimes); despite its origins, it is an all-American fabric that has gone from workwear to all-around sportswear use.

Tweed: Rough surfaced fabric with mixed color effects, often seen in checks and plaids. Originally made in country homes near the Tweed River between England and Scotland.

Poplin: Fabrics with a fine imbedded rib including cotton, silk, wool, blends or man-made fabrics.

Seersucker: A lightweight cotton or cotton-blend fabric characterized by an alternating crinkled, puckered stripe and a smooth stripe running vertically. First woven in India, the name comes from a Hindi corruption of a Persian phrase "shir shakkar" which translates as "milk and sugar" referring to the rough and smooth texture.

Silk: A luxury fabric made by a silkworm in forming a cocoon. It is elastic, resilient and strong while being very lightweight, and it absorbs dyes extremely well.

Brushed Cotton: Cotton or cotton-blended fabrics which are brushed to produce a slight nap and softness to the finish.

Polished Cotton: A tightly woven group of cotton fabrics characterized by a sheen, ranging from dull to bright, which produces a dressier cloth compared to most other cottons.

Linen: Made from the flax plant, linen is a lustrous and cool fabric guaranteed to wrinkle. It is easily recognized by its characteristic slub and beautiful colors.

Cotton Twill: One of the three basic weaves (satin and plain being the other two), it is identified by its diagonal rib running upward from left to right. Very sturdy and common, it is available in all cotton and cotton-blends.

A MATTER OF PLEATS

I firmly believe four things about pleats:

- Pleats are a matter of function, not fashion.
- Anyone, young or old, can wear pleats.
- Anyone, heavy or thin, can wear pleats.
- Pleats reduce wrinkling across the lap.

There are two types of pleats:

- Forward Pleats—These are sometimes called English pleats and open toward the zipper at the front of the pant.
- Reverse Pleats—This style is currently more popular. They open toward the pockets or rear of the pant.

By their very nature, pleats have a fuller thigh portion of the pant leg than the plain front models. If you absolutely refuse to try a fuller leg trouser, you cannot wear pleats—either forward or reverse.

The main difficulty in trying pleats for the first time is the feeling of too much fabric in the hip and thigh area whether or not there actually is. Mostly it is a matter of getting used to seeing a different silhouette when you look in a mirror.

I have seen every size and shape of man wear pleats successfully with only one point of guidance: Pleated trousers are meant to be worn on your waist not your hips. (Wearing them too low causes a baggy effect in both the hips and thighs, not welcomed by men who are already heavy in this area.) Worn correctly, pleats can actually be slimming, especially when secured by braces. They form a long vertical line running up the leg to the waist thus creating an illusion of slimness.

Here are some truisms about pleated trousers:

- They are cooler in warm weather since they are looser and allow more circulation.

- When you sit down, your hips expand and the pleats expand right along with you.
- If fitted properly, they are slimming.
- Pleats have been and will continue to be in style for a long time.

TO CUFF OR NOT TO CUFF

Beyond some common sense guidelines, the decision of whether or not to wear a cuff is a matter of personal choice. Most people feel that cuffs are more conservative/dressy, and therefore would be out of place on a pair of golf slacks or, more obviously, a pair of jeans. A sleek, European-style suit with a pair of beautiful Italian leather shoes would not be consistent with cuffs. The opposite would be true of a fine English or American business suit with a classic cap toe shoe. Here, a cuff would be elegant and perfectly in place.

There is some debate as to whether cuffs are appropriate for a short man. Cuffs do provide more weight and pull to anchor the pant bottoms and make them drape properly, this forms a long vertical line using the crease and the pleat to create the illusion of a longer leg line. I believe in the end it is a matter of personal choice.

If the decision of cuffing is to be based on camouflaging, here is a simple guide: To elongate the leg, choose cuffless pants; to minimize long legs, choose a cuff .

The width of the cuff is not a very serious issue. As long as it isn't so wide as to look like you were accompanying the Duke of Windsor through a walk in the muddy fields and trying to protect your trouser bottoms or the other extreme of a slim, little sliver which is hardly worth the effort, you can't err too much. A rule of thumb is about one to one and one-half inches.

A WORD ABOUT TROUSER CROTCH LININGS

For some men, the crotch of their trousers wears out too quickly. Heat and friction wears away even the most expensive wool fabrics. It has nothing to do with the fabric not holding up well. This condition can be patched but not fixed. It is far better to prevent it by having the tailor add a layer of fabric, usually a piece of acetate or other very tough, slick material, to the crotch area. This is one of the most cost effective alterations you can have done when purchasing a pair of trousers whether separately or as part of a suit. It can often double the life of a pair of pants.

POCKETS BOWING OUT

We all have an age that we sort of think of ourselves as being. It may be 21, 25, 30, 35, or whatever. I truly feel that this is perfectly natural and harmless. Many men seem to want to do this with their pant size as well. This causes disaster.

If a few extra pounds have crept onto your waistline, which is where it seems to go on men, there is no way to wear your old pants the way they were meant to be worn. It produces what I refer to as the "ice cream cone effect," thin tapered bottom bulging to roundness above.

Before you reach this point there is a warning period. If you watch for it, you may be able to take action before you get too far out of hand. When you look at yourself in the mirror, look at the front pant pockets especially closely. Regardless whether they are on seam, diagonal or horizontal, they should lie close, fairly flat to the material on the edge of the opening, touching. If the pockets bow out, the pants are trying to compensate for slightly more than they were meant to hold. Don't fall for the trap of wearing too snug pants, expecting them to provide inspiration which will result in lost weight.

Lose the weight or have them let out. Or buy a pair of "fat pants" to wear until you can wear the smaller size.

HORIZONTAL CREASES ACROSS FRONT

A certain amount of room is built into a man's trousers so that he can sit and bend and stoop comfortably. When that built-in reserve begins to be filled up with person, it exhibits a series of horizontal lines across the lap after sitting or bending for a prolonged period of time. If the pants are made of good natural fabric, these lines will fall out in time when properly hung.

TOO SMALL WAIST SIZE

Buying and wearing a size 34-waist pant when a tape measure reads 36 when wrapped around you does not make you look thinner. It actually contributes to that male malady—the spare tire. You will actually appear thinner if your pants fit, regardless of the numbers sewn into the waistband. This is because instead of squeezing any excess up above the waistband (I've never seen anyone squeeze it down) you simply cover it and your pants can ride in the proper position. This also allows the pant leg to fall properly.

The temptation to deceive seems universal. If we wore size 34 five years.ago and can get into them today, then we must be in as good shape as we were then. The wearer is the only one who is ever fooled. The fact that the pants' waistband is worn three-and-one-half inches lower than it used to be is conveniently overlooked. A glance downward to where the cuff used to gently break as it just touched the shoe's instep, is now a cascade of material bagged up like an elephant's ankles. If time and gravity have taken their toll, then the only thing short of exercise and diet is to go up in size.

WHAT TO LOOK FOR WHEN HAVING TROUSERS FITTED

Trousers should fit at the waist. Unlike jeans that fit at the hips, trousers need to sit on the hips to provide the support that keeps them in place. The most important variable to be aware of is the rise (the distance between the base of the crotch and the waistband). The rise can vary from one manufacturer to another, so do not compromise. You cannot be comfortable if the rise is incorrect for your body type.

- If you choose to wear braces (suspenders), allow an extra half-inch in the waist to accommodate the "hardware"—the buttons and pigskin tabs.
- Belted or side-tab model trousers should be just snug enough to stay up. Insert one finger between you and the waistband to ensure comfort.
- Pockets and pleats do not bow open or pull apart when standing erect.

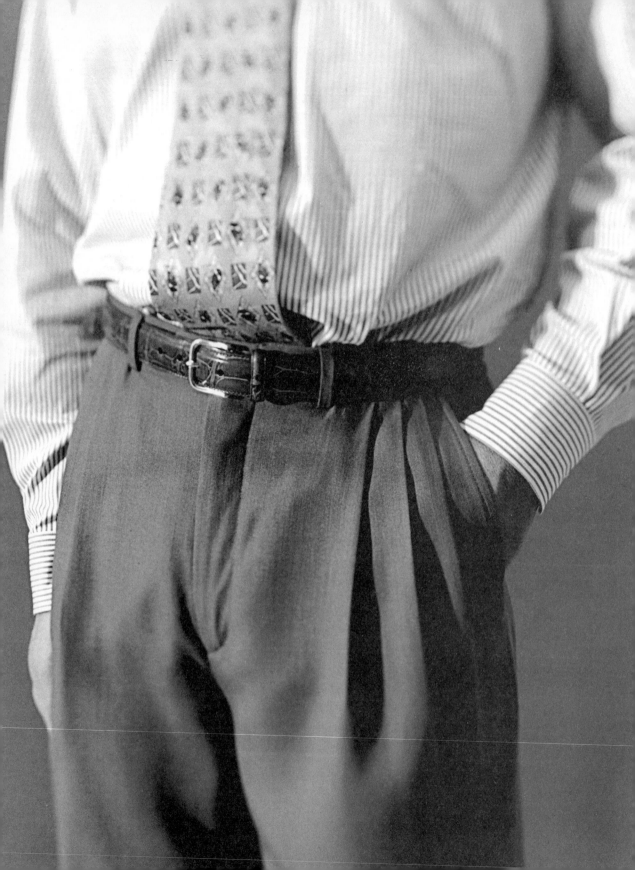

- The trouser seat may be altered to fit looser or more snugly. But be careful: These alterations usually also affect the fit at the crotch.
- Pant bottoms should "break" at the shoe tops. Avoid the two extremes of "high water pants" and "elephant ankles." High waters mean the bottoms don't reach the shoes. Elephant ankles means folds of fabric that billow over the foot. The correct length is a bit more than just touching the shoe tops. A safe rule of thumb is: Trousers must be long enough to cover your socks when you walk.
- Cuffs, should you choose to wear them, should be about one-and-a-half inches wide. Cuffed bottoms should be hemmed straight across. Uncuffed bottoms should be hemmed about one-half inch longer in back. It is always dangerous to let down a cuffless trouser leg because it is difficult to get rid or the line where the previous hem was ironed in. It's suggested that if you must lower a cuffless bottom, convert it to a cuff thus camouflaging the previous hemline.

✖ ✖ ✖

Costly thy habit as thy purse can buy,
But not express'd in fancy; rich not gaudy
For the apparel oft proclaims the man.

—William Shakespeare
Hamlet

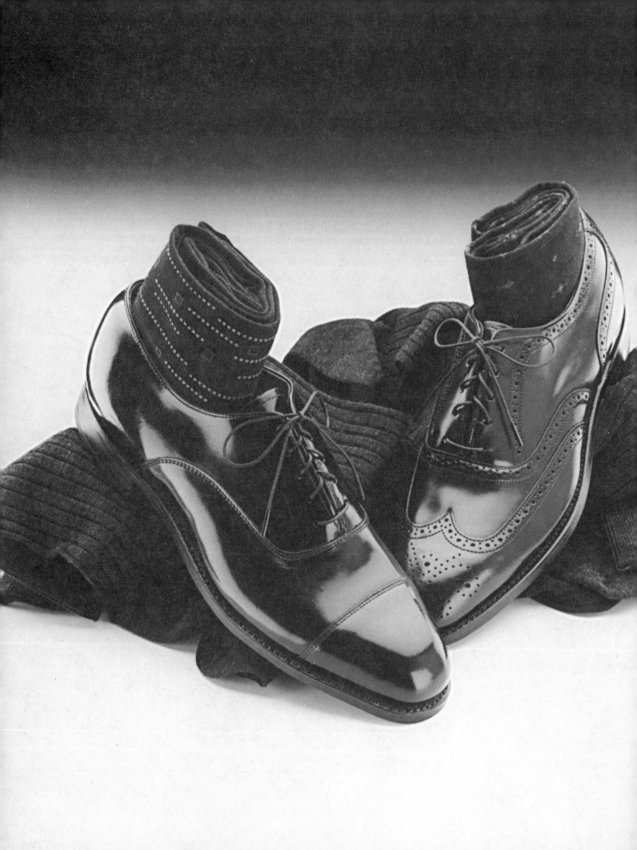

8 | Down to the Toes: Shoes and Socks

It is said that if you want to know if a man is truly well-dressed, "look down." Below the perfect break of a man's perfectly made trouser cuffs are his shoes, and if they're out of synch with the rest of him, his overall style will end abruptly. The rules tend to be painfully hard and fast: Your shoes must be right. Quality must be excellent. Fashion must be minimal. Style must be quietly and elegantly right for the occasion. Period!

Of course, there's a good deal of latitude outside the office—everything from high-tech sports shoes to the patent leather pumps of a royal coronation. Still, shoes simply must fit the moment.

It is a false economy at best—foolhardy at worst—to scrimp on your footwear. When it comes to spending a few extra dollars for the best quality, don't hesitate. You won't invest in flaky penny stocks if you're after a high-quality portfolio, and shoes are one of the highest values in any serious clothing collection. You won't regret it.

HOW TO BUY SHOES

Men's shoes are one of the best values around today, dollar for dollar. With proper care they will last for years. Periodic replacement of soles and heels, along with regular polishing with both a cream and a wax polish, and, finally, regular rest periods with a pair of good shoe trees in place will allow you to amortize the original price over many years. All the care in the world will not help if you do not make certain your shoes fit you in the first place. Here are eight tips to help you get a perfect fit.

- Shop after you have been out and about a bit, since feet do swell. This way you will get the most realistic measurement.

103

- Shop only at a store that uses a Brannock foot measuring device for determining your exact foot size.
- Almost everyone has one foot larger than the other, usually it is the right foot; fit the shoes to the larger right foot. Do not rely solely on the size you have always worn. Different makers can vary significantly from each other, even though the numeric size is the same. Buy them by how they feel on your feet.
- Allow a half-inch between the tips of your toes and your shoes. If the toes of the shoes are pointed, be certain there is enough room for your toes to move comfortably. Shoes should never be tight over the instep or ball of the foot.
- When considering an oxford-style shoe, you should not be able to tie the laces so tightly that the two edges of the shoe meet. If you can, then a narrower size is probably better for you.
- Buy leather shoes. Though more expensive, because it is porous, leather is the best for the health and comfort of your feet. In leather shoes the foot can breathe, discouraging the build-up of bacteria.
- Shoes should fit from the moment you try them on. Do not accept the salesperson's, "Once you break them in they will be fine." The man-made materials used today do not stretch significantly, but leather adapts to your foot shape quite well.
- When shopping, wear the same type of sock you will use with the dress or sports shoes. Too heavy or too thin socks will distort the fit.

QUALITY UPKEEP

A professional shoe shine is worth much more than what you pay for it.

- If you're after a winner's style and you've invested good money in your shoes, it's really unbecoming to be shy about a professional shine.
- If you are nervous about getting a professional shine for the first time, take it from me, the men shining shoes in hotels, airports, train stations or street corners are some of the friendliest people I've ever

met. From the minute you sit down in the chair they will take care of everything with gentle, knowing taps or touches. Just be friendly and enjoy the experience.

If you're the do-it-yourself type, here's a step-by-step guide to getting the kind of shine a military drill instructor would approve of:

✖✖ POLISHING SHOES TO PERFECTION

- Cream polish such as Meltonian Cream feeds fine leather and keeps it supple. Wax polish like Kiwi Wax Polish which brings up a shine and is somewhat water resistant, will also do a good job. Both polishes come in a wide range of colors.
- Before polishing be sure to remove all dust and surface dirt. You'll need a cloth to use with cream polish, and for wax-type polish, a small circular brush for application and a separate larger one for the actual polishing will do the job.
- When polishing you may prefer to leave your shoe trees inside the shoes, providing a smoother and more stable surface to work with.

The following method is used by a number of military institutions as well as shoe shine professionals:

- Apply polish to one shoe with an applicator. Allow it to soak in while you apply a coat of polish to the other shoe.
- Wrap the corner of a clean cloth around your first and second fingers. Twist the rest of the cloth into a spiral and tighten the section around your fingers. Hold onto the spiral in the palm of your hand.
- Dab the cloth lightly along the surface of the polish.
- Rub the polish into the toe in a circular motion. As the surface dries out and the cloth begins to drag, spit lightly on the shoe. (If you've been eating or drinking sweets or dairy products this can become messy. Instead, use a spray mister or put a few drops of water in the lid of your polish container and dip the applicator in that.)
- Continue to add polish, a little at a time, and cover the entire shoe.

- Very lightly buff the shoe with the polishing brush (most of the best are made out of horse hair). This will bring out the shine, so don't press too firmly.
- Finally, using a soft clean cloth, rub briskly back and forth to bring out a high luster.

THE VALUE OF SHOE TREES

There is little debate about the value of a pair of good wooden shoe trees. The best are made of cedar and they do so much for such a small investment. The average man produces up to a half pint of perspiration per day and most of it is absorbed by the leather lining and uppers of the shoe. Shoe trees draw the moisture away from the leather allowing them to dry more efficiently and to retain their shape. Also, by discouraging bacterial build-up, shoe odor is kept in check. Many experts claim that the average man would double the life of his favorite pair of shoes by simply putting a pair of shoe trees into them as soon as he took them off at the end of the day.

SEVEN PRIMARY SHOE STYLES WORN IN BUSINESS

Cap-Toe Oxford: The cap-toe is the dressiest and most popular of all the business shoe styles. This shoe has been the backbone of the well-dressed businessman's wardrobe both here and abroad. It is identified by a plain toe separated from the rest of the shoe by a thin band of leather either plain or with perforations running along the strip; it looks best when worn with the more serious suit fabrics and styles. Available in various shades of black, brown and cordovan, regional differences in acceptable colors have developed. In some areas, the dark brown version is considered proper to wear with a navy suit, while in another area, it would be considered in poor taste with anything but an earth- toned suit of olive, brown or tan. Black is fine with all of the serious dark colors of gray and navy but not at all with any of the earth tones. Cordovan is the one color that seems to go with everything and is understood everywhere.

Medallion/Perforated Cap-Toe: This model of shoe is very similar to the cap-toe; the most significant difference is the amount of decoration formed by an arrangement of dots or perforations. The entire toe piece is covered with a perforated design as is the stitching that runs along the saddle of the shoe. This model is just slightly less dressy, but can be worn with the standard suit fabrics such as worsteds and flannel. Because of the decoration, it does not serve as a substitute formal wear shoe the way a plain cap-toe might.

Wing-Tip Oxford: The wing-tip is heavier than other models and is quite easily identified by the large amount of decoration (various sizes of perforations) covering the shoe. And, instead of a straight band of fabric setting off the toe, you will find a sweeping design running from toe to mid-shoe which resembles the wing of a bird. Because of its texture and heft, it can be worn successfully with the more textured and heavier fabrics like tweed, flannel and even cheviots.

Plain-Toe Oxford: As the name implies, there is no decoration at all on the toe piece, just a perfectly smooth expanse of leather that should be highly polished. Acceptable in all business situations, the only caution is when a perforated band of saddling is added for decoration. This addition makes the shoe become less dressy and certainly not a formal wear substitute, especially if the black saddle is paired with a different color of leather such as cordovan.

Monk Strap: This enduring classic is a plain-toed, side-buckled shoe of European design. It is most commonly made of calfskin, but brown suede leather is very popular with the man who would like a touch of uniqueness in his dress footwear. It can be worn for occasions ranging from fairly sporty to very dressy depending on the overall effect to be achieved by the outfit, the suede model being generally considered less dressy than the polished or pebbled surface calf-skin.

Dress Slip-On: Everyone can tell the difference between a lace-up and a slip-on but the line separating a dress or casual slip-on is murkier.

SHOE STYLES

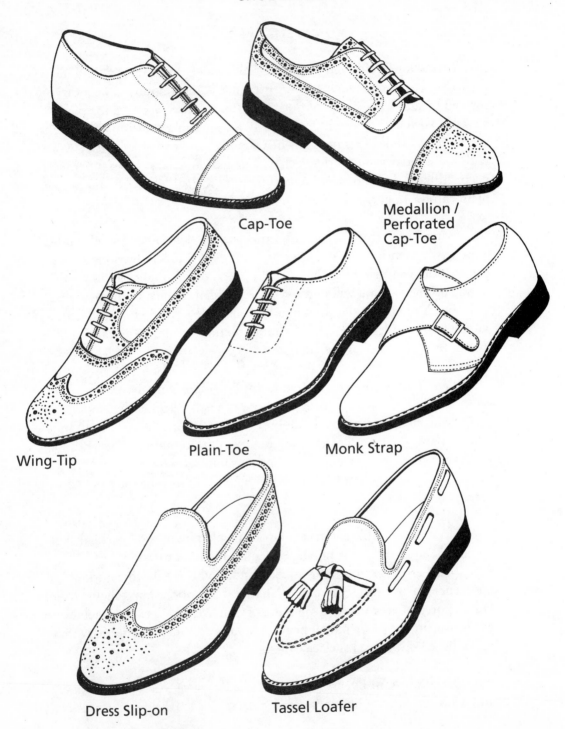

Cap-Toe

Medallion /
Perforated
Cap-Toe

Wing-Tip

Plain-Toe

Monk Strap

Dress Slip-on

Tassel Loafer

There is no one feature to look for when trying to decide; the overriding consideration is appropriateness. A sleek, lightweight European-style shoe with gold or silver ornamentation would be perfectly at home paired with cotton khakis and a short- sleeved knit shirt but is too informal to wear with a traditional business suit. A dress slip-on with the basic toe detailing of a cap-toe, medallion or wing-tip will provide the needed formality while still providing the comfort and convenience so much in demand today.

Tassel Loafer: The black tassel loafer has been around since the twenties and, if anything, has gained increasing acceptance as an appropriate business shoe. Now commonly seen in not only black but also brown and the reddish-black color referred to as Bordeaux, burgundy, ox-blood or cordovan.

Cordovan is widely used to describe a color but is technically a type of waxy, long-wearing material that comes from the hindmost quarter of a horse. It contains almost no pores, is resistant to water and can be polished to an exceptionally bright shine.

WHAT A DIFFERENCE A SHOE MAKES

Casual shoes are an important element in completing an outfit chosen to be worn for less dressy occassions. You cannot look well dressed if you try to get away with wearing your business footwear with tan cotton or interesting plaid pants. Of the many styles available the following will let you combine form and function.

Loafer with Low Vamp: Because of its low vamp, kiltie or decorative hardware, this loafer does not fit the description of a proper business shoe. However, men are wearing it with business suits all over the country, especially in large urban areas. Less conservative occupations such as advertising, retailing, sales and the garment industries are the most accepting. Men in conservative occupations such as banking, government, law and medicine will probably choose to save this style for casual outfits.

Reebok/Rockport Dress Shoes: Essentially this is a shoe that evolved for function not fashion. The uppers look like any other conservative dress shoe in all of the acceptable colors. The major identifiable feature is the sole, which is a thicker, softer version made of "rubber." It provides comfort and a cushioned step. It has been remarkably well-received in all walks of life where large amounts of time are spent on one's feet. Those who stand a lot or must walk long distances in hallways or airport terminals sing their praises.

Sueded Leather Oxfords: We are talking about the suede cap-toe with a dress leather sole that can be worn with the most sophisticated business outfits. It was introduced by the Duke of Windsor, who was among the first to take this shoe out of the country and pair it with a business suit. The look is one of sophistication and confidence.

Penny Loafers: This is the most widely recognized casual shoe around. Traditionally, a penny was put inside a slit in the leather band that runs across the instep. Either the standard or modified version (which includes a tassel on the band) are very correct with almost any form of sportswear.

Moccasin-Style Slip-On: This is a slip-on shoe adapted from the Indian moccasin made from one piece of leather sewn over a vamp. They come in a wide range of colors and fabric types, and the soles can be soft, firm, Vibram™, or rubberized with little nubs on them.

Rugged Lug-Soled Oiled Leather: A treated leather upper which is almost impervious to weather. The sole is very rugged looking and thick. They come in both slip-on and lace-up models and are generally found in various earth tones such as bark, olive, brandy and so forth.

Boat Shoes with Rubber Soles: This once strictly functional piece of footwear has become very popular. They're great for boating because the leather uppers resist soaking while on the water and no matter how wet they get, they dry to a loving softness with no special attention. Their soft, white, smooth soles are perfect for traversing wet surfaces safely without danger of scratching or marring the polished teak deck of even the finest yacht. Sailors of every age, whether aboard a dingy or 52-foot ocean racer, wear these shoes as an indispensable part of their sailor's outfit.

Bucks: An old standby among lace-up shoes for summer wear, the white buck comes with a red rubber sole or Nu-Buck™ in shades of brown, tan or buff and can be worn year-round.

Chukka/Desert Boots: This is a high-cut shoe that extends a little over the ankle and is usually made of calfskin or suede and always seems to remain in fashion. It is usually fitted with a cushy rubber sole making it a great walking shoe. In addition, it provides a great deal of support for walking on uneven terrain.

Rubber/Gum Soled Moccasins: Made to stand up to the most severe weather, this injection molded shoe is usually seen with dark brown rubber uppers and cream colored lug-soled bottoms. It was adopted by the equestrian set because of its easily cleaned construction. Many have a removable felt sole liner for use in cold weather.

Aqua Socks: Another injection molded shoe, this one is more like a rubber slipper. Originally intended for use while wind-surfing, it has found a place anywhere there is water—stone covered beaches, rocky water bottoms, hot pool decks as well as for use in jet-skiing and power boating. The most common colors are basic black and blue with neon bright designs and trim.

Sandals: This style of shoe is as varied as any in the world—from its cutout leather uppers to its wide variety of soles ranging from leather to rubber. Depending on the material, it is worn in many parts of the world as the standard footwear or in its all-rubber "flip-flop" version around the pool or health club locker room.

Reebok/Rockport Walking Shoes: These shoes have carved out a niche for themselves by being neutral in styling and constructed to be orthopedically sound.

Cowboy Boots: The classic version of America's contribution to footwear began as one of function: Pointed toes allow for easier slipping into a stirrup and a built-up heel prevents it from sliding through the stirrup. The toes can be pointed, square or rounded; the height can range from mid-calf to knee-high; the top can be indented or cut straight across; and they can be plain and simple or elaborately tooled leather or made from the exotic skins of ostrich or reptile. They are the perfect companion to the other American casual standby—the blue jean.

Espadrille: A rope soled beach and sports shoe with canvas uppers, originally worn by Spanish and French dock hands. This is a light, comfortable shoe designed to be worn without socks. The canvas uppers come in a wide range of colors.

DON'T FORGET THE DETAILS

The following thoughts will make you a "shoe-in" for having style when it comes to footwear:

UNPOLISHED SHOES

Anyone who walks around with shoes that look as though they were buffed-up using a brick and a Hershey bar is telling the world they just don't care. Not a pretty picture. Not caring bespeaks an attitude that has no place in the business or professional community. So our message is: Keep a shine.

GUNBOAT-STYLE SHOES

A special note to recently separated military types: The Armed Forces issue a good quality, long-wearing shoe to its personnel and it is easy to think of it as an acceptable piece of civilian wear after separation. Not true. Don't fall into this trap. A proper pair of business shoes should have a sole with a thickness of 5/8" or less. Look at the stitches on the top of the sole. The most expensive, as well as most familiar, method of attaching the sole to the uppers is referred to as the Goodyear welt. It is a grooved effect that runs around the shoe. Usually, inexpensive or sporty shoes won't use this method. Of course, few people will carefully examine your shoe's soles, but you'll know.

Check the inner lining and the uppers, both of which should be leather. Top-quality cowhide and calfskin are good choices, as is cordovan. Avoid most man-made fabrics and anything that looks as though small planes could take off from them.

✖✖ DRESS SHOES AND CASUAL ATTIRE

Avoid making mistakes in this area by learning what goes with what. Shoes that are at home with a business suit should not be worn with jeans, casual pants such as linen blends or ducks, and most positively not with Bermuda shorts.

Slip-on shoes present a minefield full of potential problems when worn with a suit. There is a tasseled loafer seen in the business community on stockbrokers, retailers and people in the clothing industry. It is considered an acceptable look for these and other non-conservative occupations, yet only a top-quality cowhide or cordovan model will do. The economy models just don't cut it.

- Penny loafers are best not worn with suits. Youngsters can pull this look off, but it usually is considered improper—shoes like penny loafers, Topsiders, and most slip-ons belong with slacks and open-collared sports shirt or even a sport coat and tie.
- Athletic shoes have a clear-cut place. If you are ever tempted to wear your Nike's with your suit, the way that many young female professionals have, don't do it.

✖✖ BOOTS WITH A SUIT

There is such a thing as a Chelsea dress boot but few men know about them and fewer still own and wear them. We will not discuss them here. Chukkas, desert boots and cowboy boots do not have a place in a business setting, unless you are mapping out the lease area of your next oil and gas venture in the Oklahoma Panhandle.

✖✖ ALLIGATOR NIPPING AT YOUR HEELS

A recent poll revealed that one of the major differences between men and women and how they rank important items of apparel, is in shoes and their maintenance. Some women complain that they have no shoes to wear while surveying 75 pairs sitting nearly untouched in their original boxes. A pair for every conceivable occasion except, of course, the one they need to be shod for at the moment.

Conversely, a man will own a total of three pairs of shoes and try to make them work with everything. The problem arises as his business pair begins to wear down. He knows that having them repaired will leave him without them for about a week. Because he has an important meeting scheduled for the middle of the week, he puts it off until the following weekend. This goes on and on until he comes upon a "While-U-Wait" repair shop, usually by chance. Don't let this happen to you. If you can put your shoe on a flat surface with the eraser end of a pencil against the heel and the eraser fits under, they are in need of repair. Replace the heels once in a while; it's a very cost-effective way to make them last.

✖✖ THREE COLORS OF MEN'S DRESS SHOES AND COORDINATION GUIDE

Black: Goes with black, of course, but also with navy and almost every shade of gray. It does not go with any shade of brown, olive or tan.

Brown: Is best suited to all of the various shades of "earth tones" available today. Dark brown, tan, olive and taupe pants or suits are perfect when paired with either calf or suede shoes in any of the shades of brown.

Cordovan: This reddish-black color seems to go with almost everything from navy, cadet blue, gray to all the earth tones. If you do a good deal of traveling, this is a good choice since it will go with so many different outfits.

SOCK IT AWAY

First, a story: I was once called upon to assist a retiring major general in making the transition to civilian clothing. We selected the appropriate suits, shirts, ties and shoes for his pending interviews. After a couple of hours of selecting and fitting, he breathed a sigh of relief and said, "That was good and not nearly as painful as I feared. About the only thing that leaves me with are my black G.I. socks." To which I responded, "Well General, let's talk about that for a minute." I took him over to the socks pointing out the desirability of considering some new, updated patterns as options to his old black, nylon "friends." After agreeing to give them a try, he left the store with his purchases.

A week later, the general returned and summoned me from across the room— as only a general could do—with a precise left-face complete with heel click as he marched to the sock display. When I caught up with him, he said "I got complimented on my new socks everytime I wore 'em." "That's great," I said. "But," he continued sternly, "I never got a compliment on my socks before in my life!" I looked him straight in the eye and asked "What were people supposed to say to you—nice black?" He laughed and added, "Well, I liked the feeling of getting compliments—so let's try some more, OK?" To this day he still comments on how surprised he was that such a small change could produce such noticeable results.

It's true, though. As "small" a style matter as updating your socks seems, the impact of this often-neglected apparel can be quite significant. Yet many men continue to play it safe with black socks and wear them with everything. With a dark colored pair of pants as part of a business or dress look, they're no problem. But gentlemen, buy some different socks to wear with your corduroys, Bermuda shorts and all of your favorite colored sports clothes. Jeans and black socks don't mix!

SOCK PATTERNS FOR DRESS AND CASUAL WEAR

In addition to color, of course, there is enough variety in sock patterns to appeal to everyone. Here are the main design patterns:

Bird's-eye: A woven or knitted small, rounded pattern of two or three colors with a small center dot resembling a bird's eye.

Nail's Head: A small dotted design resembling the rounded effect of a group of flat head nails arranged in overlapping fashion.

Paisley: Printed or woven designs of abstract, curved shapes that resemble a number of different things depending on your imagination—an amoebae orgy, fish swimming in a pool or the seed of a fig tree. (The pattern, according to one of the many theories, was derived from the palmette motif of Persian rugs.)

Houndstooth Check: A checkered design with uneven edges resembling the teeth of a dog.

Cable-Stitch: An overlapping knit stitch simulating a twisted rope design or cable; the cable is generally the same color as the rest of the sock.

Argyle: Any multi-colored knitted diamond pattern on a solid color background. (Not related to or derived from the Argyle Clan in Scotland.)

Herringbone: Sometimes called a chevron weave, a fabric in which alternating rows of thread slant right and left forming a pattern resembling a fish's skeletal system.

Neat: Any plain woven fabric with a pattern of small, evenly-spaced designs covering the entire surface.

A FINAL NOTE ON SOCKS

Regardless of what pattern or colored sock you choose, there is still one cardinal rule: NO SKIN SHOWING WHEN SEATED. It's not an attractive sight. Despite this well-meaning advice, men still find themselves inadvertently exposing their hairy/semi-hairy shins to the world. Whose fault is this? More than anything else, it's due to modern science. Before the perfection of man-made elasticized socks, silk, cotton or wool socks really had no way to stay up on a man's leg. Garters were used for this purpose. The arrival of socks with an elastic band around the top was a God-send. Men streamed to the "Black Sock Store" in droves to pick up a dozen pairs of jet black socks and then forgot about them until the socks one by one began to disappear in the clothes dryer which signaled another trip to the "Black Sock Store."

Not much of a God-send, was it?

For comfort, they were made shorter, as the synthetic band cut off circulation to some people's legs. Then came all-synthetics, which had elastic mixed all through the sock. The length remained fairly short—not over the calf—again because the fabric didn't breathe and was uncomfortable. They stayed up fine but the problem is that you can't seem to kill them— they last forever. So if you are waiting for them to fall apart before replacing them forget it! Wash them repeatedly, bake them in a dryer, they just never seem to need replacement. But replace them you should! If you can't remember when you bought them, consider seriously buying a pair of new state-of-the-art socks. The difference will amaze you. They stay up and they are comfortable since they contain a large amount of natural fiber.

✖ ✖ ✖

Boots and shoes are the greatest trouble in
my life. Everything else one can turn
new; but there's no coaxing boots and
shoes to look better than they are.
—George Elliott
Amos Barton

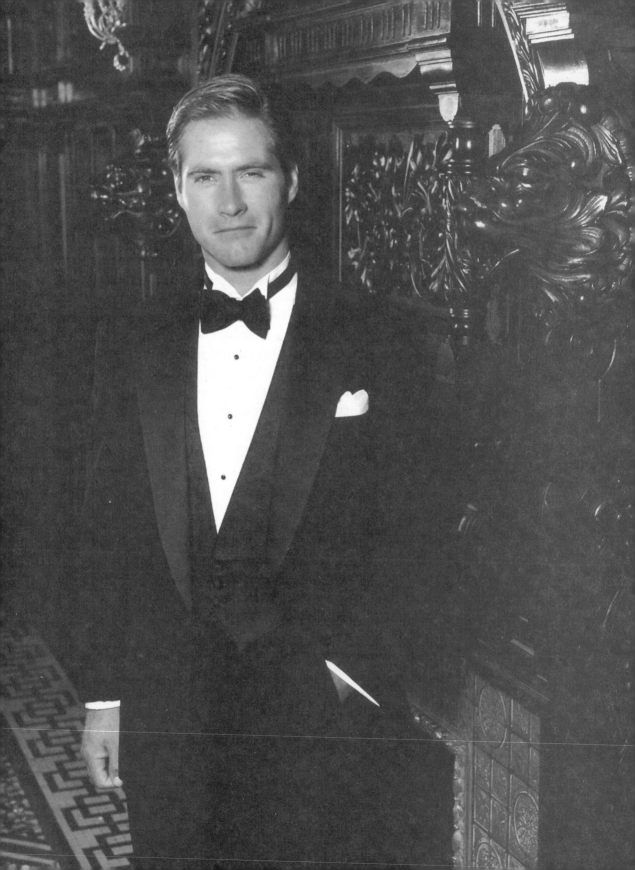

9 | Non-Business Style: No Tie to Black Tie

During the course of most business careers, opportunities will present themselves requiring dress ranging from everyday business attire to black tie to no tie at all and each is as important as the others when it comes to creating and preserving your image. Most men have clothing that is suitable for painting the house, cutting the grass or just lounging around, and they have adequate clothing in which to go to work. But many have absolutely nothing in between these two extremes.

Today, the line between business and pleasure is razor thin. Never before has what you choose to wear in pursuit of seemingly non-business activities been so important. The proliferation of invitations from colleagues, clients and senior management calling for the dress to be "informal/casual" has created countless situations that have never been discussed in any detail before. Each situation can be a boon or a bust as to how people will perceive you long after the "informal/casual" occasion has passed.

The first thing to recognize is that a successful, responsible person is expected to look that way regardless of the activity. Showing up looking vastly different than people normally see you is not in your best interest. If your usual attire is a suit, white shirt and tie with black cap-toed shoes, do not show up at the company picnic dressed in your high-top red sneakers, cut-off denims complete with holes and a Grateful Dead World Tour T-shirt; it confuses people and forces them to wonder which is the real you.

Casual wear presents the opportunity to display a little personality and individuality; and staying within the bounds of good taste is both essential and really pretty easy if you simply see to it that you have a variety of pieces that fall into the category of sportswear. True sportswear that is, not simply the same blue shirt you would normally wear to the office but leaving off the tie and rolling up the sleeves.

119

What follows is an ideal closet from which you should be able to select items that are appropriate to be worn during a number of activities while still being comfortable and respectable.

SOME SUGGESTED CLOTHING ITEMS TO HAVE ON HAND

FALL/WINTER

Shirts—

- Cotton turtleneck in a variety of colors
- Cotton/wool flannel country shirt, plaid or print
- Viyella (wool and cotton blend) long-sleeve
- Traditional oxford cloth button-down
- Rugby shirts
- Corduroy long-sleeve-solid/pattern
- Denim long-sleeve

Sweaters—

- Shetland crew neck
- Cable knit crew or V-neck
- Sleeveless sweater vest-wool or wool/cashmere blend
- Cashmere cardigan or V-neck
- Irish Fisherman's sweater
- Wool separate vest, solid or plaid

Pants—

- Blue jeans washed and faded and pressed but no holes
- Pleated gray flannels
- Tan cavalry twill—wool
- Navy mid-weight wool or blend
- Corduroys, nail's head, fine, medium or wide wale
- Cotton tan twills
- Plaid or houndstooth checks
- Warm-up pants

Sports coats—

- Flannel or year-round navy blazer
- Cashmere sports coat—any color or plaid

Jackets—

- English oiled-cotton shooting jacket
- Suede leather hip-length baseball style
- Distressed leather bomber jacket
- Poplin windbreaker with knit collar and cuffs
- Down-filled vest
- Weather-resistant hooded parka windbreaker

Shoes—

- Penny loafers
- Suede oxfords
- Chukka boots
- Hiking shoes, lightweight over the ankle
- Cowboy boots
- Kiltie-tassel loafers

Accessories—

- Plaid wool or cashmere scarf
- Deerskin gloves w/liner
- Knit stocking cap
- Irish walking hat

✖✖ SPRING/SUMMER

Shirts—

- Cotton madras button-down
- Short-sleeve cotton lisle
- Cotton "polo" style pique or interlock
- Linen—short sleeve
- Woven prints

- Hawaiian print in cotton or rayon
- Woven cotton shirt with a knit collar
- Oversize cotton broadcloth cover-up (white with emblem or monogram)

Pants—

- Cotton ducks in tan, navy or olive
- Cotton khaki twills
- Rugby shorts
- Bathing trunks, trim boxer style
- Plaid walking shorts
- Navy, tan and olive Bermuda shorts
- Tropical-weight wool dress trousers

Sweaters—

- Cotton crew neck
- Boat neck sweater
- Cable knit cotton tennis or cricket style pullover
- Sleeveless cotton pullover
- Cotton sweatshirt

Jackets—

- Lightweight safari style
- Ten-month cotton "drizzler" (Barracuda™)
- Nylon windbreaker

Shoes—

- Oiled leather boat shoes
- Espadrilles
- Casual slip-ons
- Suede bucks
- Leather cross-trainers
- Lace-up walking shoes

Socks—

- White sport socks
- Ankle-length bicycle/walking socks
- Calf-length tennis socks
- Variety of blend or cotton patterned socks

Accessories—

- Woven leather or colorful fabric belts
- Fabric madras/repp stripe watchband
- Reptile skin-type belt
- Leather belt with decorative buckle

Style Tip: Just selecting a clean pair of pants and a shirt not found rolled in a ball on the floor of the closet is not enough. Try to tie the two pieces together with a third piece such as a sweater, vest, casual jacket or layered shirt. The addition of something as small as a belt, patterned sock or watchband which coordinates with the colors of the shirt and pants will create a wonderfully complete look.

A NOTE ABOUT NAVY BLAZERS

Probably no single article of clothing can illustrate the significant differences in attitudes between a man and a woman when it comes to clothing as the navy blazer. To a female, it may be boring—nothing special. A male, on the other hand, thinks a blazer is classic, authoritative and indispensable.

After all, it has those official looking solid brass buttons, goes with lots of different pairs of pants, everyone he knows has one and looks good in it, and it is in style 12 months a year. Walking into a holiday party, a man and a woman pause at the top of the staircase to view the already arrived guests gathered below. Should the woman see even a remote duplication of her outfit, the entire evening could be dampened. But if the man glances down and sees 13 other men wearing a navy blue blazer, his first thought is "Whew! I wore the right thing."

CASUAL DAY AT THE OFFICE IS NOT YOUR DAY OFF

Casual day is a good idea that has been introduced as a way to improve morale, give employees a head start on their way to the woods or beach for the weekend, or simply because everyone agrees to relax the dress code for a day, week or month. It has promptly been rescinded in many organizations for basically one reason—people abusing the freedom to relax and taking it to mean anything goes. Anything does not go. It is still your job and the activities of business must still be conducted, sometimes even with people from the outside who have not heard of "casual day." No list of articles of apparel not to be worn could possibly cover every conceivable error lurking in your closet.

A few words of guidance along with several examples should serve to give you a good idea of what to wear without destroying your credibility within the organization.

- Clothes must be clean, pressed and in good repair
- T-shirts should not be used as a public service broadcast medium unless it is the organization's message
- Leave your necktie at home unless it is a theme or conversational tie depicting your off-duty interest
- Wear a non-traditional shirt (denim, chambray, flannel)with a string tie
- Have a blazer, sports coat or cardigan handy in case you need it for an unexpected meeting
- Jeans and a wonderfully ornate belt buckle will go with everything
- Patterned socks with chinos and a knit shirt is safely "casual smart"
- Shoes or boots should be very comfortable but be sure they are clean and respectable

One of the best overall tips I have ever heard for determining what would be considered good for casual day at the office is this: Once you have dressed, stop and ask this one question of yourself: If I were going to help a friend move into his new home or work in the garden or on his car what would I change before we got started? If the answer is nothing, you have dressed too casually for casual-day at work.

FORMAL WEAR—FOR THOSE SPECIAL TIMES

If the occasion calls for a tuxedo and you decide to rent, most of your decisions are over. The store will measure you and allow you to select from the available styles and accessories—which may or may not be to your liking. But you can really get in trouble renting a tuxedo—just take a look at those prom night parties! So take a little extra time to locate a formal wear rental store who has done a good job in the past for someone you know.

If and when you decide to purchase a tuxedo, here is some basic information to consider:

There is no "best" style. The major choice is between a single- or double-breasted jacket and that is an individual preference— use the same guidelines as in selecting a suit. Single-breasted is considered more conservative and will be safely and stylishly worn for years to come; double-breasted is more dramatic but can, from time to time, be declared "outré" by fashion arbiters. Double-breasted is warmer due to the double wrap of fabric across the front which is meant to be kept buttoned at all times.

✖✖ COLOR???

Don't even think about anything other than basic black! I agree with the dozens of women I checked with: *Most men look their most handsome when they are wearing a tux.*

The next decision involves lapel styles:

Notched lapel: This is the most common and the most conservative of all. It has a V-shaped indentation where the collar and lapel meet. It suits most every body type and has stayed in fashion for more than 100 years; it shows no signs of being replaced.

Peaked lapel: Normally this style is found on double-breasted models but I have seen it on single-breasted fronts as well. This lapel flares out at right angles to the rest of the lapel, forming two sharp points that, at their widest point, are considerably wider than the notched version. It is not quite as flattering on a smaller man.

Shawl collar: Most often seen on white dinner jackets, this collar extends from the button hole, up the front and around the neck and is rolled back without notches or peaks of any kind. This style is considered to be very traditional.

The fabric on most tuxedo lapels is usually either satin (a smooth, lustrous, somewhat heavy fabric made of silk, polyester or a combination of other fabrics) or grosgrain (a fabric of silk, rayon or other fibers along with cotton filling to produce a ribbed effect).

No store will carry every combination of lapel style and fabric. Each will carry styles appropriate to its clientele. If you have had good luck buying suits at a particular store, chances are you will be happy with the tuxedos they offer.

There are few other choices to be made in selecting a tuxedo. The fabric covered buttons on the jacket and the satin braid running down the outside of each tuxedo leg are fairly standard. Formal trousers are always worn without cuffs.

✖✖ FORMAL SHIRTS

Choose a straight-forward, good quality white cotton with simple pleats in the front. I consider the five-pleat front to be slightly classier than the busier ten-pleat. The choice of collar is between a straight and wing style. The straight is the more conservative and looks better on most men. For a more fashionable look, or just for a change of pace, a winged collar can be fun. If you choose a winged collar, place the points or "wings" behind the bow tie—the same as with a straight collar.

Formal shirts always have French cuffs, so you will need cuff links. You will also need a set of studs to replace the plain buttons that come on a formal shirt and have confused more than a few otherwise intelligent men. Studs can be as fancy or expensive as you can afford. Most, however, are made of various semi-precious stones or plain gold, either polished or matte finished, and are reasonably priced. Most often they are sold in matching stud and cuff link sets.

Studs with small round or oval backs are my personal favorite, since they tend to stay in the buttonholes best. The ones with the small bars that move up and down when inserting into the buttonholes have an annoying habit of finding their way out of the hole, leaving you with a gaping shirt front. They were originally intended to be worn with formal shirts with rounded buttonholes and a valet to help with all the details. With the advent of the current straight cut hole, (not to mention the demise of personal valets) this style doesn't work nearly as well.

✖✖ CUMMERBUNDS AND TIES

Black satin or grosgrain are always a correct choice for these two tuxedo accessories. However, the more colorful sets are fun and run the gamut from subdued colors to patterns, dashiki cloth to hand-painted one-of-a-kinds. Take into account the formality of the occasion and your desire to make a "personal statement."

There is an old maxim that the cummerbund's pleats served to catch whatever crumbs a gentleman dropped during the course of dinner—and therefore should be worn with those "crumb-catching" pleats facing up. Call me a romantic, but I prefer to think of the pleats as being the holder of the evening's theater tickets. The original dinner suit—the forerunner of the tuxedo—traditionally was designed with no pockets (well before the days of credit cards, driver's licenses, etc.) The cummerbund pleats facing up were a safe and convenient holder for the evening's absolute necessities.

✖✖ BRACES

A necessary tuxedo accessory, braces are designed to button to the inside of the trousers, thus performing the necessary function of holding up your trousers (cummerbunds are not effective for this purpose, and no tuxedo comes with belt loops). Black is the safest color choice, but by no means the only one. Since your braces will not normally be seen, you may have some real fun with them. Case in point—A very nice and normally very conservative man that I helped for years was being remarried and chose the traditional black tuxedo and conservative accessories— with one twist: a pair of silk braces adorned with little pink naked angels. When the public part of the day was over, he wanted to make a bold statement. He tells me he did.

SOCKS

Your socks should always be black. From time to time, people will wear a bright-colored pair of socks for fun at a social occasion calling for black tie (New Year's Eve, for instance), but this is an exception not the rule.

SHOES

Black, well-shined slips-ons or lace-ups will do if we are reaching the outer limit of your budget. However, for the truly finished look, patent leather pumps or four-eyed, lace-up oxfords are considered the perfect formal shoe.

A FINAL NOTE ON FORMAL UPKEEP

Try keeping your tuxedo pressed and ready to go in a plastic covering or garment bag. Put the formal shirt in the same bag if on a hanger, or, if folded, in a sweater bag with all of the accessories. Patent leather shoes should be kept in a soft cotton shoe bag to prevent scratching or gathering dust which can dull the finish when wiped off. This way, when that formal occasion arises, everything is easily found and ready to be put on. Few things can put a damper on the evening's festivities faster than a frantic last minute search for the set of studs you have not seen in six months.

YOUR WEDDING

On this very special day, you can wear anything you and your partner choose. Your choice of formal wear, either rented or purchased, should fit, be currently stylish and in good repair—the same rules apply if you choose to wear a new, special suit on your wedding day. Just remember: You will be seeing that outfit for a long time to come on your mantle, at your family's home, the home of your in-laws and friends in the wedding party. Years from now, when styles have changed, you may wish you had selected a more conservative model, color or pattern.

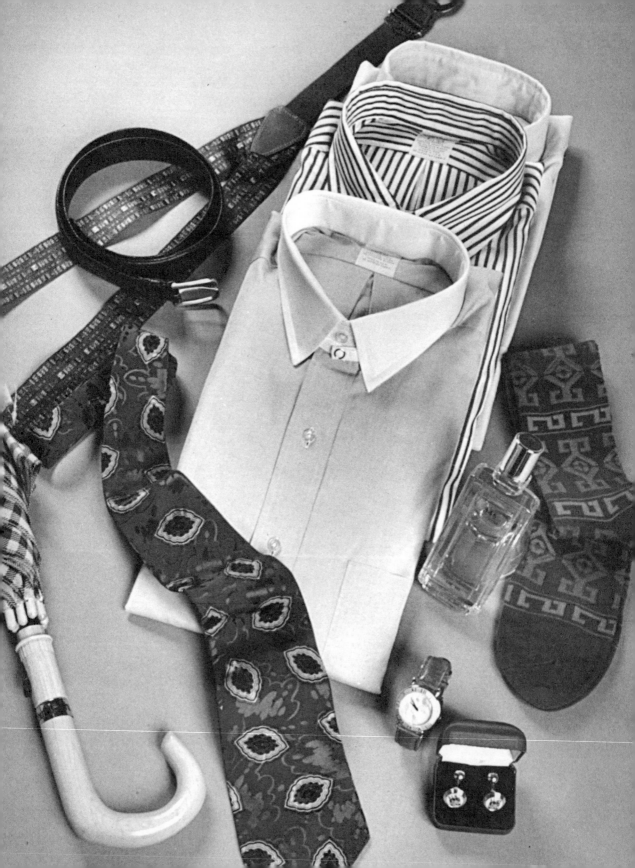

10 | Accessory Etiquette

Accessories—those casual items from pens to belts—can be the trickiest pieces of any man's wardrobe. As inconsequential as they may seem, they are the very details that make the stylish difference. Why invest a lot of time and money in your look only to allow your good work and imagination to be ruined by a leaky ball-point pen, especially since such disasters are so avoidable?

In this chapter, we'll teach you how to use your accessories to create a look that is uniquely you and how to avoid the pitfalls inherent in their use. Giving your accessories the respect they deserve will help you keep your style in top form.

 ## RULE OF SEVEN

Let's begin with a time tested guideline that will help you avoid overall clutter. It is called the "Rule of Seven." Simply stated, there should be no more than seven points of interest on your body at any time. A point of interest is anything that in and of itself draws attention. Things that might be counted as points are: collar bar, bright tie, pocket square, fraternal pin, shiny blazer buttons, braces, fashion glasses, facial hair, peaked lapels or a vest.

Researchers found that when volunteers looked at a series of pictures while answering simple questions they had no problem until the picture became more complex— seven points of interest— at which time they had difficulty answering even the simplest questions. Their attention was being drawn to the visual stimuli and they were missing the verbal message.

FAT WALLETS

Turning your wallet into a micro-version of a woman's purse doesn't work. We are not born with, nor do we inherit, a wallet the size of a Big Mac™; yet, you will see them nearly everywhere you look. A recent check of a friend's wallet revealed the following contents: an American Express corporate credit card, a magnetic card to open a garage door, a video club membership card, seven different bank and department store cards and a VIP Travel Club card. Also, an automatic teller machine card, a hospital insurance I.D. card, 27 credit card receipts, and three pieces of paper with notes on them as well as the balance of an unused note pad.

All I can say is: WRONG! Pare it down to the bare minimum for the maximum look. Each day, decide what items are necessary and leave the rest at home. Men don't seem to notice the fat wallet syndrome and what it does to the shape of the pant in the back. Wedging that mass of leather and paper into a rear pocket causes an unsightly bulge none of us need. Wallets aren't born fat; put yours on a diet!

WEARING A POCKET SQUARE

A pocket handkerchief—called a pocket square by people in the menswear business—can be quite dashing. If you choose to wear one, your tie should coordinate with it but not match. Pull out, as an accent, one color in your tie and repeat that color in your pocket square. Even the pattern can be different. A striped or foulard tie can be enhanced by the addition of a subtle paisley silk pocket square whose base color coordinates with one of the colors in the necktie.

There are a dizzying number of ways to wear a pocket square and the feeling each fold imparts says a little bit about the personality of the wearer. Since pocket squares can add so much to your total look, it is important to know how to wear them several different ways to express the feeling of the moment or be appropriate to the event.

Here are seven different ways to fold a pocket square, along with illustrations of how each should look when you're finished:

• **The Puff.** Hold the square by its center, grasp the material with your other hand about half way down. Now, insert thepoints, which should be hanging straight down, into the pocket. Spread the fabric so it fills the pocket opening and only a "puff" of fabric shows.

• **The Flop.** Hold the fabric by its center; using the thumb andforefinger of your other hand, circle the square as it hangs straight down. Slide your circling finger and thumb down a bit more than half way. Insert the square's center into the pocket allowing the points to fall freely or "flop" over.

• **The Plop.** Begin with the square completely open. Fold in half, and then in half again in order to form a smaller square. Pick up this smaller square by its center. With your other hand, gently roll all of the loose points together. Once you've done that you should be holding a roughly cone-shaped piece of silk. Push the points into your jacket pocket and arrange the pointed top so that a dimple shows in the center.

• **Four Point.** Start by folding the open square into an imperfect riangle. Next, fold up one of the lower corners so its point is separated by a few inches from the existing two points. By folding the other corner in the same way you'll have four points. Fold the base up and insert the pocket square into the pocket. Arrange the points to show all four clearly.

• **Three Point.** Fold the square into a perfect triangle. Match the points carefully. Have the flat side toward you, the top of the triangle facing away. Move the lower left corner to the right of the top by a couple of inches. Next, move the right hand corner to the left of the top. Adjust points so that they are even in height and spacing. Fold the bottom up about half way and push into your pocket.

• **TV Fold.** This is the simplest of all. Almost always done with a solid color handkerchief, it was very popular during the 1950s although it originated in the forties. When your handkerchief is folded to one-eighth its full size, just slip the side with the most edges into your pocket leaving about one-half to one inch showing above your pocket line. Be sure it's razor straight.

• **The Peaks.** Begin with the pocket square completely open.Fold over diagonally to form a perfect triangle with the flat side to your right. Fold the bottom edge up just to right of edge farthest from you and slightly

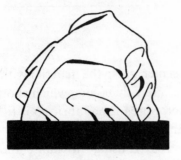

The Puff

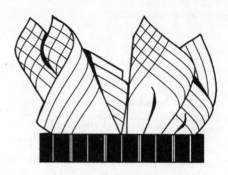

The Flop

POCKET SQUARES

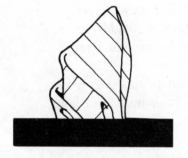

The Plop

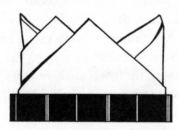

Four Point

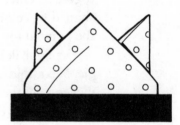

Three Point

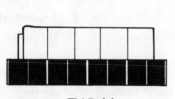

TV Fold

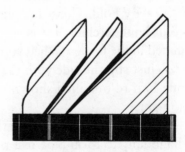

The Peaks

higher. Now move the left edge slightly higher and to the right of the two peaks at the top You should have a new triangle with the only difference of three peaks at the top. Fold point sides over to become parallel with the flat side of the triangle. Next fold the bottom edge up toward but just short of the peaks. Carefully slide the folded square into place. Adjust if necessary.

POCKETFUL OF PENS

Whether or not it is "nerdy" or "logical" to sheath 12 pens in a plastic case to protect your shirt from ink spots is really not the issue. There just isn't any reason to carry this artillery around with you. The average pen is more than capable of writing 10,000 words before giving up the ghost; very few people put even a fraction of that down on paper during any given day. If you use a writing instrument frequently for signatures, brief notes, appointments or phone numbers, limit yourself to one pen, and, if you choose a matched set, one pencil. These should be of first-rate quality. After all, if you are using them frequently, and especially if you allow others to use them in business transactions, they should say something positive about you.

If disposable pens are your current choice consider this: When you hand a person a pen at the completion of a business transaction to sign the agreement , it should feel good in their hand; the act of signing should be pleasant and smooth and convey a positive end to the process. The over-all sensation should underscore the positive feeling of the entire event. All of these good feelings radiate over to you and how you do business. That is how it should be. If a valued client uses your purchased-by-the-gross, generic pen and, while signing, either smudges or skips or, worst of all, leaves an ink stain on their first finger, the reaction will be one of UGH!, and that reaction will reflect on you as well. It will introduce a negative cloud over the whole deal. You don't need someone going UGH! at you.

✖✖ DISCREET STORAGE

For those of you who remove your jackets only while at your desks, try keeping your pen in an inside coat pocket . Many manufacturers sew in a pen pocket on the left side of the lining specifically for this purpose.

A good tailor can add such a pocket and it will be worth the expense. If most of your day is spent without a jacket on and you need a pen at the ready, the shirt pocket is not the only place to carry it. The three most popular alternative locations are:

- in the calendar/date book that you carry;
- in the right back pocket of your trousers instead of a wallet;
- clipped to the shirt placket underneath your necktie.

CAPTAIN KANGAROO SYNDROME

From childhood right on through their golden years, men exhibit a nearly perverse love of pockets. Even a sophisticated sports coat can have as many as seven of them. For some, pockets are temporary storage areas; for others, they become treasure troves, yielding all sorts of strange and wonderful things ranging from a forgotten $20 bill to the ticket stubs from last year's charity event.

Most suits come with the outside pockets sewn shut. The simple reason is that the line of the coat is cleaner without sagging or bulging pockets. If you need a little help to overcome the habit of loading things into your pockets, why not try leaving them sewn shut? Oxford Clothiers, makers of what many consider to be the finest ready-to-wear clothing anywhere, constructs its clothing with pockets that billow inward to help camouflage the Captain Kangaroo Syndrome.

Whatever can logically be carried in a briefcase should be: extra pens, breath mints, calculator, and so forth. Keep the items on your person to the barest of minimums. And use the available pockets wisely: The front breast pocket is meant to carry a pocket square or a pair of eyeglasses but not both; the outside right pocket should have a small pocket sewn in it to be used for spare change or car keys; the inside right pocket is most often used for valuables such as a wallet, passport or appointment calendar often with a flap that closes over the pocket for added security.

Several manufacturers, Joseph J. Pietrafesa among them, have created a unique feature found in suits they manufacture for a number of retail stores: The pocket not only goes down as you would expect but it is also cut going up to enlarge it and allow the flap to button over slightly larger items being carried here. The inside left pocket located down low near the skirt cut into the lining of the jacket was originally called the cigarette pocket. Lately, it has been used more for carrying a business card case or breath freshener and is terribly under used. It may seem odd at first, but, with a little practice, this handy pocket will prove to be invaluable. The left side inner breast pocket is used for a functional handkerchief. If a pen pocket has been sewn in by the manufacturer, it will be located next to the inner left pocket. An eyeglass pocket, an extremely rare option, is located just below the left inner breast pocket.

 ## NO "GORILLA-PROOF" BRIEFCASES NEED APPLY

No other accessory that a man can wear or carry says as much about him as his briefcase. Just the fact that a man is carrying a briefcase tells us quite a bit about him even before a single word is exchanged. He may be a collector of rare antiques or an oil baron. His home may be a chateau, his car the finest available, but, remember, they cannot be brought with him into a business meeting.

Think about the various types of briefcases and the images they convey. The nearly square sample case identifies the carrier as a salesman. The book-bag style case gives the impression of a scholar. A thin leather portfolio suggests its owner needs to carry very little but what he brings is of great importance. A vinyl portfolio says just the opposite. Why would the fact that your case can fall out of an airplane undamaged or be mauled by a gorilla inspire any measure of confidence in you? A fine leather briefcase in a conservative color says all of the right things about you, whether you are a new junior executive or an established old veteran. Please, if you possibly can, invest in this one item. It will be worth it. A good piece of leather, well constructed, will last for many years and will improve with age.

✖ ✖ ✖

"WATCH" YOUR STYLE

A gentleman's watch should be plain and simple, made of either gold or silver, and preferably does not have a picture of a famous rodent or political slogan on its face. Its band is made of leather, metal, non-endangered reptile skins or woven fabric (grosgrain) in a variety of colors . The more you deviate from these guidelines, the better your chance of spoiling your mature professional look.

There is something distracting about a watch that fires off signal flares and plays the first 16 bars of the "The Star Spangled Banner" to announce the hour. Mini-computer watches have a place, but it isn't in a serious, professional setting. Digitals are less formal, and can be inappropriate in a business situation.

There are a wide variety of watches that can be perfectly acceptable in any business or dress situation. Names such as Cartier, Rolex, Movado, Concorde, Piaget and Bulova, to mention a few. If your budget strains under the thought of one of these time-honored names, one company that can help is called Exactly; it creates copies of the classic watch styles for a fraction of the price. Most are not only beautiful but also classically elegant and can be found in many major department and specialty stores around the country.

CLASS RINGS WITH NO CLASS

There really is no clear-cut time to stop wearing the class ring, a symbol of so many fond memories and not a few broken hearts. But once you've seriously entered into the business world, you should consider retiring it to your jewelry box.

In today's competitive business environment it is an unwritten code that you represent your company or company's product line. Anything that identifies you as a member of some outside group or affiliation, regardless of how harmless, has the potential of interfering with normal business communications. Selling yourself or your products is tough enough without some unspoken hidden objection hanging around getting in the way. As much as you love your alma mater, someone else feels the same about his or hers.

BETTER BELT BEHAVIOR

We now turn to that old venerable friend, your belt. It's such an old friend, in fact, that we tend to take it for granted, as if it were invisible. And in business/professional settings the overall effect should be one of harmony and blending in. Dark calfskin with a discrete metal buckle is all you need.

Making an overt display of your belt (especially the buckle) forces those around you to focus on the area near your navel, often not our most flattering area and can do as much to detract from your overall appearance as a garish tie or poorly-cared-for shoes.

OVERLY ORNATE BUCKLE

Anything other than a simple gold or silver buckle is out of place with a traditional business suit. There is a lot to be said for the beautiful works of art available as clasps for sport/casual wear. They can be a terrific way to express a mood or make a statement, but you cannot, must not, try to combine a three-pound piece of turquoise or a replica of the Inca sun god with a business suit.

You may have a good haircut, handsome features, an expensive suit, shirt and tie. But if you're wearing a belt buckle that is an exact replica of a snub-nosed 38-caliber revolver, you are shooting yourself in the foot.

BRACE YOURSELF!

As clear cut as it may seem, you should always wear a belt when your pants have belt loops. There is one major exception to that dogmatic statement:

Never wear your belt with suspenders (or braces, as they are alternately called). Both belts and braces serve the same function but they do it in different ways; it's the method of support that's a matter of personal choice. Wear one or the other, but not both. Some folks remove the loops when they have suspender buttons sewn on and some manufacturers don't even include loops if the garment was designed to be worn without a belt.

Most often these will be identified by the small tab closure in the front of the pants where the belt buckle would ordinarily be found.

EYEGLASS FRAMES: CHOOSING THE RIGHT ONES FOR YOU

For some reason, there is a lot of confusion when it comes to selecting the eyeglass frames that look best on you. Sometimes we pay more attention to fashionable or trendy designs or new eyeglass materials that are in vogue, than to the actual materials used in the frames. Are they a color that goes with your eyes and skin tones? Do they go with the shape of your face? The most expensive or chic frames on the market will look awful if they don't compliment your face. Study yourself carefully in the mirror, decide which of the face shapes describes you best, and make your selection based on the following proven points:

• **Round:** A round faced man needs to create the illusion of having cheekbones by selecting frames that are straight across the top, angle inward toward the bottom, which is also straight across. Round frames and curved ones should be avoided as they will accentuate the roundness of your face. Stay away from very square styles; they will create too much of a contrast.

• **Square:** Slightly rounded or curved frames with height on top can modify a square face. Aviator frames often look very good especially if you're young or have stayed in good shape. Your goal is to select a shape that will lengthen the look of your face.

• **Rectangle:** When we refer to this shape we mean long and squarish not short and wide. This shape needs to add some width. A wide, square frame with slightly rounded corners or overall rounded styles seem to create the best look.

• **Oblong:** The oblong face is long but doesn't have the square-ness of the rectangular. Your goal is to add both width and angles. Select slightly wide frames with rounded sides and straight bottoms to add shape. Choose largish glasses with heavier sides.

• **Diamond:** The diamond face needs to create the illusion of wider

EYEGLASS FRAMES

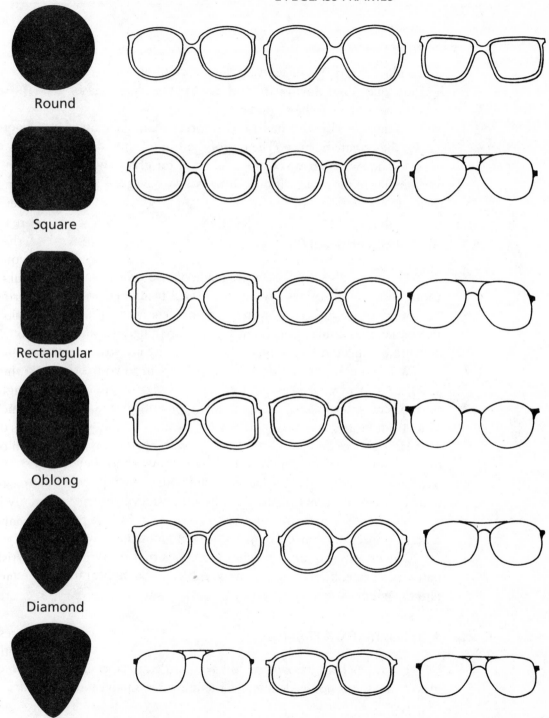

Round

Square

Rectangular

Oblong

Diamond

Triangular

chin and forehead. You need frames with width on top, straight sides, and bottoms that point downward and outward, such as aviator glasses. An oval frame is likely to be a good choice.

• **Triangle:** This face has a broad forehead and narrow chin. Choose glasses that create balance. The top of the frames shouldn't be heavy and the sides, not wider than your temple. Look for glasses with a curved bottom, similar to the aviator frame. Keep away from square shapes and styles with a heavy bridge.

MATERIALS AND COLOR

The materials your frames are made of also project various messages about you. Metal frames say "utility." Old-fashioned wire "specs" say "serious." Tortoise-shell or horned rims are "classic." Clear plastic frames are special; they tend to go with just about anything, and, at the same time, they project function and utility. Their versatility is a strong, selling point.

When it comes to color, you should key in to your skin tone, hair and the color of your eyes. Women use pastel, milky, or barely frosted rims to achieve a romantic look. For men, romantic just doesn't work. Stay away from pastels and trendy colors. On men, they look foppish.

Half-glasses are flexible and can go with almost any look, provided the packaging is right. Thin metal half-glasses work to project an expressive look. Heavier metal half-glasses blend with straight hair and fit in with most business uniforms. Tortoise-shells are businesslike.

Silver trims and frames are for cool coloring. Gold is for clear, warm tones. Coppery or bronze-like metals go with muted and warm skin tones.

The essential point is to choose frames that harmonize with your natural coloring. It is the surest way to enhance your appearance and maintain the winner's style.

A QUICK TAKE ON FRAMES

For the person who wants to have a little guidance in selecting eyeglass frames, but not as detailed as the information given above, here are five tips:

1. Frames should not overpower your facial features. A thick, dark plastic frame can set up a barrier to effective communication. To be comfortable with you, people need to see your eyes, and when they cannot, they can distrust you without really knowing why.

2. Eyeglass frames should not create a second eyebrow above your natural eyebrow. This look is almost extraterrestrial; it has been known to frighten little children.

3. As the name implies, the frame should frame the eye. The pupil sitting in the center of the frame makes eye contact easy and natural.

4. Frames that are small in proportion to your face project a natural look, a down-to-earth feel. Proportionate frames—where the amount of glass above and below the eye are nearly equal—are more classic in style.

5. "Aviator" frames or larger frames say "fashion." Women can get by with fashionable frames; for a man, it's much harder. Unless you're in a creative field where expressive attire is acceptable, stick to the functional frames of high quality.

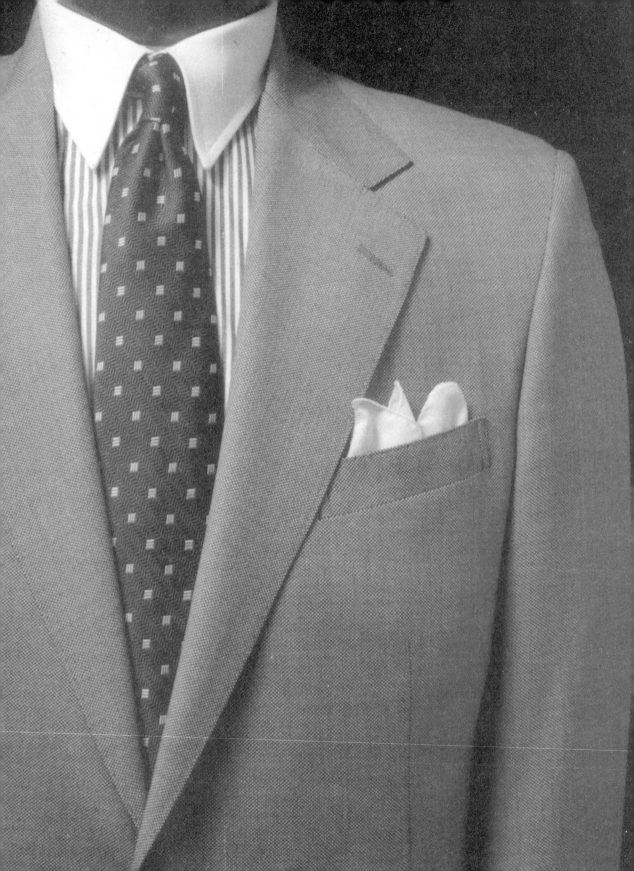

11 | Your Guide to Perfect Grooming

We all know people who do everything right. Their clothes are always the latest styles, cleaned and pressed. Their attitude is always positive and burning the midnight oil is normal for them. Every hair of their flattering hairstyle is in place. They would never think of dancing 'til dawn on a work-night for fear it might impair their work.

You may or may not be one of them, but in a business situation looking good can most definitely overcome a multitude of sins. The boss isn't interested in your headache or your aches and pains; he or she wants your appearance to reflect positively on the company. Sure, you went overboard a bit at last night's party. But today you've got to close a deal, and you've got to project the kind of poise and confidence and smile that makes the client feel smart doing business with you. It's just good business.

Your suit, tie, shirt and shoes may be perfect—and that much is expected. Still, there's another side. Your hair, face and hands They are often the better half of winning someone's respect and trust. A stain on your tie is certainly not a point in your favor, but the man or woman on the other side of the desk is likely to overlook this small human error if your grooming says better things about you.

Here are some step-by-step guides to make your grooming easier:

HAIR TODAY

It's safe to say that the male "looks revolution" was pulled into the current decade "by the hair." The decline of the age-old barber shop and the spectacular rise of the men's hairstylist was a precursor of today's preoccupation with the winner's style.

Balance means that the hair is properly cut to match facial structure, that it compliments one's looks as much as any article of clothing or point of grooming. You should feel as good about your hair as you do your suit The corporate look is "together"—all together! Everything about you, including hair, should be clean, neat and.styled correctly You shouldn't have to think about or fuss over it. Hair should be as natural as anything else about a man. It should have a look that says, "the hair takes care of itself."

✖✖ HAIR COLOR

Men are coloring their hair these days, which was heresy only a few years ago. The new attitude goes along with today's heightened awareness. Most coloring is aimed at grayness—getting rid of all or part of it. Gray at the temples is still acceptable to men, but premature graying isn't. The prime consideration is the avoidance of the "dyed look." This radical changeover isn't part of the corporate environment, which requires stability from top to bottom. If you are going to color your hair, do it very slowly. It should be gradual, so that no one really notices it.

As for doing it yourself, be careful. Many over-the-counter dyes are harsh and damaging. The gray you're trying to get rid of may just fall out if you fail to get the advice of someone who knows which formulas are effective and safe.

A few other tips from the pros:

- If you use a blow dryer, be aware that a high heat setting can play havoc with your scalp and hair, drying both. Keep the heat setting minimal.
- Use a good moisturizer on hair and scalp to reduce any possible damage.
- Men tend to shampoo more than women. Lots of shampooing can also dry your hair and scalp, so use a good conditioner.
- If your scalp is naturally dry, use a shampoo with a light moisturizer in it such as jojoba oil. It's also healthy for thin hair.

- An oily scalp can stand additional drying agents. Again, check with a pro before you cause chemical havoc.
- Normal hair—neither too dry nor oily—needs only a good cleanser. Don't bother with fancy (and fanciful) ingredients.

✖✖ HAIRSTYLES

Most men are lost when it comes to choosing a hairstyle for themselves. They feel a hairstyle is something they were born with and must maintain for the rest of their lives. Their favorite words when settling into the stylist's chair are, "Same as last time" or "Just a trim, please."

Every good haircut must be styled to the individual. To do that you must pay attention to two key elements: the shape of your face and the type and texture of your hair.

First, determine your face shape:

- **Round Face:** The objective of the cut is to narrow the face. The sleek look of the hair cut evenly in length all around and brushed back from the forehead with only a partial or no part is preferable. Sideburns, if you choose to wear them, should be on the short side (above the middle of the ear). Brush them back or have the stylist trim them at a very slight angle. Stylists recommend height on top, and hair a bit longer in the back for a taller look.
- **Long and Narrow Face:** A rounder style of haircut, with hair a bit fuller on the sides and longer in back, since you need a cut that adds width to your face while maintaining your long neck. Keep sideburns very short (to the top of the cartilage point in the ear).
- **Heart-Shaped or Triangular Face:** The goal if you have a broad forehead and narrow jaw is to balance the face; too much hair on top just emphasizes the narrowness of the jaw line. Clip the hair in layers on the top and the sides. Sideburns should be about one-half-inch below the top of the ear. If the face is narrower at the forehead than at the jaw, a round-type hairstyle, one with a longer, fuller side can help. The idea is to fill in thin temples and de-emphasize the jaw line.

• **Square Face:** For men this is an excellent face shape. Keep the cut you choose fairly short all around. Since you will look good in just about any cut, discuss with your stylist accentuating one of your finer features: eyes, jaw or cheekbones. Sideburns should be slightly on the long side (below the cartilage point).

• **Oval Face:** Many people consider this the best of all possible face shapes. You can wear just about any style successfully. Try it short on the sides and long in front, vary the length of your sideburns. Don't feel you have to stick to one look. Talk to your stylist about a style that can be worn conservatively during the day and "let loose" for a night on the town.

HAIR TEXTURE

You don't have much freedom when it comes to your hair's texture and type, but here are a few suggestions that may help:

• **Thick, curly hair:** should always be kept on the short side.

• **Fine, straight hair:** a short cut will keep it more manageable. If you choose to wear your hair longer, then you must learn to blow dry it properly, using a good natural bristle brush and a styling attachment.

• **Thinning hair:** should always be cut short, no matter what your face shape is. This makes the hair look fuller. Keep your sideburns short to avoid a lopsided look—never let your side hair grow long and comb it over the balding area.

FACIAL HAIR

With rare exception, facial hair doesn't work well in business situations. On the other hand, for those willing to be meticulous and who really prefer to wear facial hair, it can be a terrific way to strengthen strong features or minimize weak ones. Depending on your face shape, hair can sometimes be used to create an illusion, much the same way that women use makeup to highlight or disguise certain features. For instance, a medium thick, wide mustache will help broaden a thin face, while a closely trimmed beard, shaped at an angle, will help make a round or wide face look much slimmer. But, if you are one of the many men whose beard is a different color than your hair, you're probably wise to avoid beards and mustaches.

✖✖ DANDRUFF

Dandruff, which is usually associated with an excessively oily scalp and white flaking, can often be confused with something as simple as dry scalp. Several friends who thought they would never be able to wear a navy blazer found that frequent washings followed by a good conditioner worked wonders. In certain climates or during the winter months when dry heat is prevalent, a good adjunct to washing and conditioning is to use one of the many hot oil hair treatments available in stores for at-home use, or from your hair stylist or barber. If you choose to try one of the many fine home products, here is an interesting idea: Apply it while taking a leisurely steam or sauna bath.

If the problem is dandruff, a qualified dermatologist probably will be your best advisor. While dandruff can't be cured, it can be controlled. And, for those occasions when a small snowfall does occur, a good clothes or lint brush is worth its weight in gold. In a pinch, wrap adhesive tape around your hand with the sticky side out and brush lightly. Keep hands away from your head. No scratching...you may cause an avalanche!

✖✖ UNBALANCED LENGTH—LONG BACK, NO FRONT

When it comes to compensating for lost hair, men can be incredibly creative. However, allowing the hair at the back of the head to grow long is not the way to make others think you have lots of hair. It simply doesn't work! Keeping your hair length proportional to the amount you have will present the best possible look at all times.

If you have lots of hair, wear it as long as is proper for your profession. Blow dry and style for the best looking effect. If, on the other hand, you have precious little hair, take care of it and pamper it. After all, it's all you have!

✖✖
✖✖

✖✖ TOO LONG

The time for a man's hair to cover his collar in back or completely conceal his ears has passed. The look was a product of the seventies.

Men, being for the most part very conservative, want to stand back and take a wait-and-see position on most matters that have to do with dressing or grooming. The inevitable result is that some men wait until a trend or acceptable fashion has just about ended before they adopt it. Then they walk around for years thinking they really look up-to-date. Some men think that wearing their hair long somehow compensates for the thinning they wish wasn't happening. It doesn't. It makes them look like they have long, thinning hair.

The current business climate demands a neatly trimmed moderate to short length, keeping all hair where it belongs—on top of the head, not down the back or resting on the shoulders.

✖✖ COMBING EXTRA-LONG SIDE-HAIR OVER THE TOP

This is one of the most difficult ideas for many men to accept, but, allowing the hair on the side of the head to grow to extreme lengths and then combing it in the reverse direction of its natural growth over the top and over to where the other side begins simply doesn't work. It doesn't look like you have a full head of hair, and worst of all is being caught by a gust of wind that blows the hair back to the way it naturally grows. While wearing a hat outdoors works for awhile, you have to take it off, then what? The exact same thing happens when you emerge from your favorite swimming pool, lake or ocean.

If you've lost hair, or are in the process of losing it, accept it. It doesn't make you look old or bad. Most men's hairlines recede a bit, so why not blend into the crowd? Toupees or transplants work, if you must. But they have drawbacks: Toupees slip. Transplants hurt.

✖ ✖ ✖

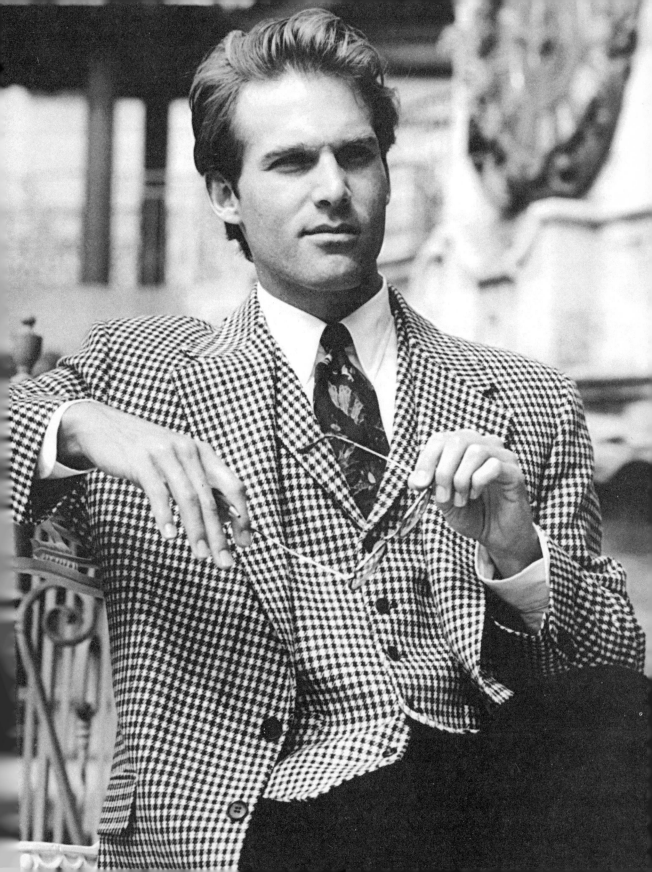

POORLY GROOMED HANDS

A man's hands are on display virtually every minute of the day. Handing a report to a secretary or colleague, pointing to a column of numbers, shaking hands and eating lunch are activities that spotlight the very area that most men studiously avoid paying proper attention to each and every day. The reason for this is not because men felt it wasn't important. As a matter of fact, of the hundred or so men we talked to, all agreed on the need for clean, well-groomed hands. But only two had ever received a professional manicure—one by a girlfriend and the other on orders from his company (his hand was part of a photo to be used in the annual report).

The mystique of the "manicure" seemed to be the culprit behind most men's reluctance. What to expect from a manicurist? First, she will cut and shape your nails to the proper length. Notice that she will cut your nails corner to center, other corner to center and center across tip. Next is a soak. The position of your hands is a little awkward for most guys but it only lasts about five minutes. Then, using an orange stick, usually with cotton over the end, she will gently push back your cuticles. Finally, she will gently buff your nail beds, always going in one direction. Never back and forth. Resist the well-meaning suggestion to have clear polish applied. It is just too shiny. If you want or need a little something, see if a light top coat won't suffice.

All you need is a once-a-month visit to supplement your at-home care—a paltry 20 minutes out of the 43,200 minutes available every month. If you aren't sure that this effort has tangible results, or feel that you do a "good enough" job with your trusty pocket clippers, do a little experiment: try a professional manicure. The first time you go, have only one hand done and commit to fairly judging the difference. It will be so startling you may not believe your own eyes. If you're still unsure about visiting a manicurist, the following will help:

✖✖ DO-IT-YOURSELF MANICURE

Some men think of their hands as working objects, as "tools" that are expected to be a bit scuffed and soiled. That's fine if you work out- of-doors. But in today's corporate environment a workman's hands—which on a true outdoors man are proud symbols of honest labor—just don't make friends. We may not think it's fair, but it's a fact.

There's another factor at work when it comes to your hands. A lot of men think it's "prissy" to fool with their fingernails. But, no longer is a manicure just for women. A part of good grooming in a business setting requires well-cared-for hands. You can grouse all you want to, but at some point you've got to accept it and do the best you can. After all, you're not alone and you know that deep down inside a manicure does not a light-weight make! Your nails grow about a quarter-inch every 10 days. If you don't want to have a professional manicure done, you can do it yourself rather easily. Tools needed: nail clippers, small scissors, an emery board (not metal), an orange stick (that's what color it is), a pumice stone (for removing rough spots), a hand lotion (used to soften and moisturize), a nail buffer (for finishing touches), a small bowl with warm water and a capful of mild dish washing liquid (for soaking and cleaning).

1. Wash and dry hands thoroughly.

2. Use clippers to shorten the nails (clip from right to center, then left to center, finally across the top to avoid splitting).

3. File briskly with emery board in one direction only. Do one side toward the center and then the other. ,

4. When your nails are smooth and nicely rounded, place them in the soapy water for about 5 minutes. If you have stains or dirt, now is the time to gently brush them away. This also softens the cuticle and prepares you for the next step.

5. Use an orange stick to gently push the softened cuticles back over the base of the nail. Don't cut!

6. Rub the pumice stone gently around each of your nails, removing dead skin. Put your hands back into the soapy water for a few min-

utes, then under cool running water. Dry your hands thoroughly and apply a few drops of hand lotion, massaging it into and around the nails. Finally, in a brisk motion, buff your nails to a soft gleam, but don't get them too shiny.

 ## SKIN CARE

For some reason, men don't think much about their skin. They should, since it's the most visible part of the body. It needs cleansing, exercise, rest and proper nutrition just like the rest of you. Like a winning smile, your skin mirrors your health and way of life. Here are some basic tips that will help you look fit and healthy:

1. Always cleanse your skin with lukewarm water. Using extremes of temperature can be harmful. Very hot water, for instance, opens the pores dramatically and brings subcutaneous oils to the surface. Years of this kind of action can increase oiliness, enlarge pores and permanently stretch out their elasticity. Cold water will roughen your skin as much as repeated exposure to Arctic winds.

2. Invest in "smart water"—either distilled or natural spring water. You can drink it and wash with it, making it good inside and out. These waters have fewer chemicals and salts, and your skin truly appreciates this touch of kindness.

3. Stimulate your face. Give it a mini-massage. Stand in front of the mirror and make faces at yourself. It's a form of exercise that tones the facial muscles and heightens color. All forms of exercise will help promote skin tone and a healthy complexion, but don't forget to make those funny faces a few times a week. It needs only a few minutes to bring excellent, long-lasting results.

4. Feed your face. But feed it the proper foods. If you're taking in a lot of cell-withering sodium chloride (ordinary table salt) you'll develop wrinkles at an early age. Caffeine in excess will do the same, and an

excess of refined grains and sugars can produce spots. The best nutrients are rich in Vitamin A and Vitamin E. Honey used externally will help regulate moisture content. Proteins, enzymes, minerals, collagen, RNA, elastin—there's a vast assortment of helpmates out there. Go to your local health food store and ask questions. The results can be startling.

5. Think prevention. If you're a smoker, you should be aware of a study by Dr. Harry W. Daniell which relates smoking to crow's feet around the eyes. Once you hit the 40 to 49 age bracket, he says, you are likely to appear as wrinkled as a non-smoker 20 years your senior! Over-exposure to the sun is another wrinkle causer—or worse. Recent studies indicate substantial increases in skin cancer among those who just can't seem to get enough tanning. Take the sun in small doses, moisturize with products containing aloe vera and Vitamin E and adequate sun-block.

✖ ✖ ✖

"Things have certainly changed in this country over the
last two decades. Prior to that, being overly concerned
with clothes was thought to be highly
suspect—appearance, their hair, their bodies and
their clothes. Of course this has been true in Europe
for decades. It is not considered odd for a man
to go to his barber two or three times a week
to keep up his appearance."
—Bill Blass

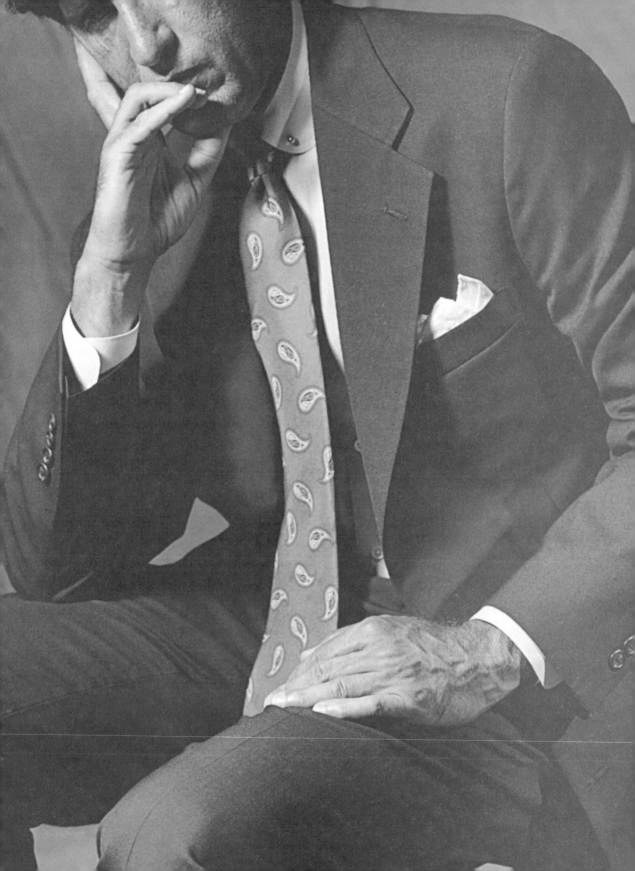

12 | Advanced Male Maintenance Skills

The very same man who treats his automobile as if it were just an extremely expensive erector set can sometimes be the same gentleman who treats his clothing as if it were an alien invader from outer space. This isn't always the case—but too often it is. Could it be that many men know more about the complex innards of their BMWs than they do about sewing on a button? Painfully, the answer appears to be yes!

There are all sorts of reasons put forth to explain this phenomenon.

Sociologists point to America's "love affair" with their automobiles.

Psychologists say men gravitate toward gadgets and leave the buttons to women. Chauvinists of the male variety speak gruffly of "woman's work," while the female counterparts insist that men don't have the tactile abilities required to properly handle needle and thread.

In the end, all sides may have valid points to make. But it doesn't solve the problem, and, meanwhile, men keep showing up at the office literally at loose ends. If you're one of these unfortunate souls, that's a shame. Chances are you won't get much in the way of sympathy from your male colleagues, and the women who want to "mother" you only reinforce your lack of skills.

So, let it end here! What follows are a lot of little tips that will go a long way toward putting your loose ends back in shape, where they belong. They add up to yet another component of the winner's style.

SEWING ON A BUTTON

Buttons are always popping off of garments at the most inconvenient time—while preparing for a major meeting with the top brass, or a thousand miles from home in a hotel room thirty minutes before a presentation to a very important client. Unless you travel with a personal valet, there will be times when having this basic repair skill will prove invaluable.

When you come across a loose button, try to figure out where it came from, as it's always easier to sew on a button shortly after it falls off. If this isn't possible, have a box or bag set aside where orphan buttons can wait until the garment-sans-button is located. If the button is lost and replacements must be purchased, here is some technical information you'll need.

Button size is measured across the diameter in "lines," 40 lines to the inch. Most of the buttons used on a suit (the sleeves, lining pocket, vest front, trouser fly and back pocket) are 24 line buttons. The jacket front is usually a 30 line button. Horn or dull bone buttons are your best bet with a classic suit of fine material. Mother of pearl or synthetic buttons are most common on shirts. Today many fine manufacturers sew a few extra buttons to the tail of their shirt fronts in the event emergency repair is necessary.

Once you have the button, you'll need a one-and-a-half-inch-long needle with a medium-sized eye. Needles are divided into sharps and betweens. Betweens are generally shorter and stronger. Sharps are medium to long in length. In both categories the needle sizes are numbered. The higher the number, the shorter and thinner the needle. A #7 sharp should take care of most repairs. Choose a color of thread that matches either the thread on the other buttons or that closely matches the color of the garment.

Mercerized cotton thread #0 or #00, or size A silk thread is suitable for most sewing jobs.

To thread the needle, cut off about a foot of thread and wet one end to help create a point. Push the thread through the needle's eye and pull it through. Tie the two ends together. If you have trouble with this, a needle threader helps.

Position the button on the garment and, starting on the wrong side of the fabric, push the needle through a hole in the button. Push the needle back through another hole in the button. Sew in an X-pattern if it's a four-hole button; make parallel stitches in a two-holer. After about six stitches, wrap the thread around the button stalk, push the needle back through the fabric and secure with a few small stitches across the back of the new button. Cut off any excess thread and, viola, you're done.

✖✖ MISSING BUTTONS

I am not an unsympathetic person. I really feel badly for the guy who puts on his last clean shirt, goes to his car and while turning his head to back out, pops a button. Usually, it is the collar button. No amount of tie tightening will conceal it. The spread of your collar will be affected and people will know that your top button isn't buttoned. They won't know if your neck is too fat to allow your shirt to close or you've just lost the button or you're a slob who just doesn't care.

If you use a commercial laundry, they will very often replace a missing button for you as part of the service. If you do not, check for loose or cracked buttons before you toss your shirt into the laundry basket. "A stitch in time saves nine," applies here, too. Many hotels provide miniature sewing kits consisting of a few buttons, a needle and variety of threads to help their guests who find themselves in need. Such a kit should be part of every man's travel kit and also a part of his "junk drawer" at the office.

If the idea of sewing is alien to you, at least try to be creative until you get your shirts back from the cleaners, out of the wash or whatever. I remember meeting with the president of a cosmetics company. In the course of the afternoon we removed our jackets. He was missing a button on his left sleeve cuff. The cuff was being held together by a safety pin. If he had a little more style, flash or "je ne sai qua" he should have pulled or cut off the button on his other cuff and pinned them both. People may have thought it was a new style of cuff link.

STAIN REMOVAL

It never hurts for your next door neighbor to be a professional dry cleaner. In the event that he is off sunning himself in St. Tropez, however, you should have a few household chemicals handy for emergencies. You should be able to deal with most problems if you have access to the following:

- Liquid dishwashing detergent
- Clear, non-fragranced ammonia
- Peroxide bleach (be careful to test on a non-visible part of the clothing—it could stain)
- White table vinegar
- A commercial enzyme presoak
- A liquid grease solvent

There are a few very common "solutions" that are used for a variety of cleaning situations. They are:

- **Enzyme solution:** one-half teaspoon of detergent diluted in one quart of warm water. (In special circumstances, which will be noted, use a quart of warm water with one tablespoon of presoak detergent solution).
- **Ammonia/detergent solution:** same as the enzyme solution with the addition of one tablespoon of ammonia.
- **Vinegar/detergent solution:** same as the enzyme solution with one tablespoon of vinegar added.

✖✖ FOOD OR PERSPIRATION STAINS

Through his necktie a man has the opportunity to express some small part of his inner self without going too far from what most of us consider conventional attire. It would be a shame to mar this statement by walking around with sweat or spaghetti sauce all over it.

The obvious solution is to have your ties properly cleaned and avoid accidents. It is, at times, impossible to prevent something from landing on your tie while on its way to your mouth. When the inevitable does happen, I suggest two ways to deal with this problem:

- Keep an extra shirt and tie in a box in your car or office (depending on where your normal work day finds you).
- If, for some reason, this idea is not possible and you must face the prospect of being seen by others with a synopsis of your lunch on your tie, you may as well point out that you've had an accident.

It has been my experience that most people are very sympathetic and will actually pay closer attention to your face or presentation!

✖✖ REMOVING STAINS IN WASHABLE GARMENTS

You will have much more success removing soil from your washable garments than your non washables. The following list is a mini-bible that will help you handle the most frequent problems:

Alcohol, Coffee, Tea, Soda: gently dab with ordinary tap water; if this doesn't do, go to a detergent solution. If you have a particularly stubborn stain then go to a detergent and ammonia mixture. If after all of this there is any remaining stain, use a little peroxide. Beer responds very well to soaking for one-half hour in an enzyme solution.

Ball-point pen ink: dab with solvent. Rub with soap and wash if the stain is still there. Sometimes spraying hairspray on the spot, allowing it to dry, then brushing it off will do the trick, too.

Blood: ordinary tap water (always cold) should be tried first. If this doesn't work, try the detergent and ammonia solution. A drop or two of peroxide should help clear up any final traces.

Catsup/Chocolate: dab with dry solvent first, let dry. If the stain remains, try a detergent solution and after that a detergent/ammonia solution if necessary.

Cosmetics (including lipstick): dab with cleaning solvent.

Fruit juice: sponge the area immediately with cold water. Dab with white vinegar if you don't discover the stain until it has dried. If necessary, presoak and wash.

Grass stains: dab with solvent and let dry. Next, soak in a detergent and vinegar solution Use peroxide for particularly stubborn stains.

Mustard: scrape off excess mustard carefully and dab with a cleaning solvent or powder. When stain persists, dab with detergent/vinegar solution.

Pencil: rub gently along the grain of the fabric with a soft eraser. If this doesn't remove the marks, wet the stain with detergent, adding a few drops of ammonia if necessary.

Alcohol: soak immediately with club soda and rinse in water.

REMOVING STAINS IN NON WASHABLE GARMENTS

Alcohol, Coffee, Tea, Soda: dab with vinegar and rinse.

Ball-point pen ink: dab with solvent. If the spot remains, send it to the dry cleaner.

Blood: a few drops of ammonia should do the job.

Catsup/Chocolate: wet the stain with a solution of one-half a teaspoon of presoak and a half-cup of warm water. Let it stand for a bit before you rinse with cold water.

Cosmetics (lipstick): if a quick application of cleaning solvent doesn't clear it up, it must go to the dry cleaner.

Fruit juice: try cold tap water first, then white vinegar if the stain has dried. If this doesn't work, then you have no choice but to send it to a dry cleaner.

Grass stain: sponge on a cleaning fluid and let it dry or you can try a cleaning powder.

Mustard: scrape off any excess mustard carefully (you don't want to spread it around) and dab with cleaning solvent or powder. Where the stain persists, dab with detergent and vinegar solution.

IRONING A SHIRT

In the best of all possible worlds you would never discover that your-favorite all cotton shirt didn't go to the laundry or your permanent pressed shirt lost its permanence. When you do or when it has, you only need access to water, an iron, a towel, a sheet or pillowcase and a flat surface.

For the most part, shirts are easier to iron when damp, not after they are completely dry. If they have dried, use a pump-spray mister to dampen the shirt as you iron. Or, put your shirts in a plastic bag in the vegetable crisper section of the refrigerator for a few hours. The combination of the cold fabric and hot iron will produce a crisp, well-pressed shirt.

Now, start ironing the yoke of the shirt and go from there to the collar, doing the inside first and then go on to the outside, pulling as tautly as you can while ironing.

Next do the back, the sleeve and then the cuffs. Iron the front last.

Begin on the button side of the shirt, iron around, not over, the buttons. There is usually an indented groove around the toe of the iron which will allow you to go around and under the buttons. When you get to the buttonhole side, be especially careful when ironing the placket—that is where the buttonholes are. The entire front should be ironed from the collar to the tail.

DO-IT-YOURSELF EYEGLASS REPAIRS

The vast majority of men have not discovered that eyewear can be used for more than correcting vision problems. Instead of considering eyewear as a piece of jewelry or an accessory, which can be used to their advantage in complimenting the skin tone and face shape, they view them as an appliance to help them see.

And, as with all appliances, men think that a little tape, a paper clip or a yard of bailing wire can fix anything as good as new. All that these short-cut fixes do is establish a fellow as someone who is clever enough to save $2.87, (which is what you'd have to pay to have a professional do the repair), at the cost of looking like a nerd.

If you travel a great deal, it's a good idea to pack an extra pair of eye glasses with your toiletries. That way, if you should accidentally sit on your glasses in your hotel room, you won't be forced to make that million-dollar presentation with a paper clip hanging down next to your temple or a roll of white adhesive tape on the bridge of your nose. If this is a recurring problem, solve it once and for all by buying a kit containing the proper replacement parts and the tools to make the repairs yourself.

PROTECTING YOUR INVESTMENT—HOW TO DECODE THE LABELS IN YOUR CLOTHES

The labels sewn inside your clothing are there as a guide to the proper care and feeding of the rather substantial investment you've made in a winner's wardrobe. Unfortunately, some of these sewn-in instructions, especially those from foreign countries, seem written for experts in Sanskrit. One day we'll have uniform, easy-to-understand instructions sewn into all our clothing, but until that fine day arrives we have no choice but to decipher the often cryptic codes the various men's clothing manufacturers have handed to us.

The symbols shown below turn out to be basic puzzlers. Here's what they're telling you:

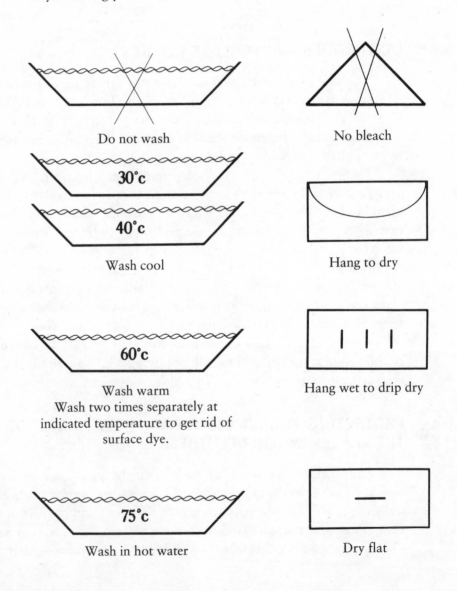

Do not wash

No bleach

30°c

40°c

Wash cool

Hang to dry

60°c

Wash warm
Wash two times separately at
indicated temperature to get rid of
surface dye.

Hang wet to drip dry

75°c

Wash in hot water

Dry flat

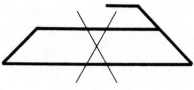

Do not iron

Do not dry clean

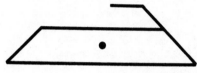

Iron low or low steam setting

Dry clean

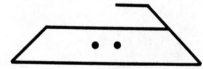

Iron medium setting

Dry clean, but not with trechlorethyl-
ene type: usual cleaners "perc" fine

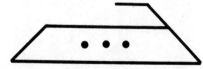

Iron cotton or linen setting

Dry clean only with petroleum or
flourocarbon solvents

Appendixes

A | The Works

The time has come to tie all of the advice together into one place. The following list is only a reference and not a rigid set of rules to be adhered to without regard to the situation, individual or unique circumstances involved. Something that works extremely well in many situations can look out of place in another and no text can possibly cover every set of circumstances. Sticking to the list of what works best will serve you well most of the time. Even in the rare instance when a special set of exceptions may cause the choice to be less than perfect you will have erred on the side of universally accepted principles, so you will never be too far off the mark.

✖✖ WHAT WORKS BEST

HEAD AND FACE

WHAT WORKS BEST	WHAT WORKS LESS
Short, conservative hair cut	Hair that can be ponytailed—unless you're a film-maker or a hair stylist
Neatly combed, clean hair	Unkempt and dirty (pony-tailed or not)
Well-trimmed mustache	Long and droopy, a la Pancho Villa
Conservative eyeglass frames	Tinted glasses for indoors

✖✖
✖✖

✖✖ WHAT WORKS BEST

SHIRT

Comfortably fit shirt collar

French cuffs for the office

Subtle monograms on pocket

Sleeve $1/4$–$1/2$-inch longer
than jacket

Jacket skirt covers your seat

Natural fabrics

Bone buttons, hand sewn

Patterns matched where possible

TROUSERS

Cuffed with small break

Smooth fitting seat

Comfortable fitting waistband

Well-pressed pleated trousers

BRACES AND TIES

Stylish braces

100% silk tie about 4" wide

Necktie reaching belt line

Proper use of the label loop

BELT

Simple, classic belt buckle

One-and-one-half-inch wide
leather or reptile

WHAT WORKS LESS

Eye-bulging, face-reddening tight

Flashy, oversized cuff links

Initials on collar or cuff

Sleeve much shorter than jacket

Jacket too short or too long

More than 50% man-made fabric

Plastic buttons sewn flat

Patterns unmatched at seams

Plain bottom and too short

Baggy or tight seat

Bulging waistband

Plain front with wrinkled lap

Braces and belt together

Wash-and-wear lobster bib

Tie shorter than belt line

Dated tie tacks and tie bars

Giant, ornate, flashy buckles

Any color plastic

✖✖ WHAT WORKS BEST

POCKET SQUARE

Compliments your necktie

ACCESSORIES

Simple classic watch leather band

Wedding band

Hard or soft leather briefcase

TRENCH COAT

Tan, olive or gray raincoat

Long, clean and pressed

SOCKS

Gray, navy or black for business

Over-the-calf socks

Subtle patterns for business

SHOES

Good, dark leather well-kept

Highly polished captoe oxford

WHAT WORKS LESS

Matches necktie

Star wars 12-function chronograph

Pinky rings

Indestructible plastic or metal carrier

Black trench coat

"Columbo like" trench

Black socks with everything

Skin-showing short socks

Argyles or loud colors

Cheap, unpolished shoes

"Patent-like" military shoes for important business occasions

✷✷ A CLOSET THAT WORKS

ITEMS	MUST HAVES	$ EACH	TOTAL	ADD*
SUITS&	1 GOOD SUIT	$500	$500	XXX
BLAZER	3 EVERYDAY	$300	$900	XXX
	1 BLAZER	$150	$150	
TROUSERS	GRAY,OLIVE,TAN	$90	$90	XXX
SHIRTS	1 FRENCH CUFF	$45	$45	
	7 PIN-POINT OXFORD (4-B.D. & 3-STND.)	$35	$245	XXX
TIES	10 SILK PATTERNS	$35	$350	XXX
BRACES	2 SOLID	$35	$70	
	1 PATTERN	$45	$45	XXX
PKT SQ.	1 SOLID	$10	$10	
	1 PATTERN	$20	$20	XXX
SHOES	1 BLACK	$150	$150	
	1 CORDOVAN	$175	$175	
SOCKS	3 NAVY	7@$9	$63	XXX
	3 GRAY			
	1 BLACK			
	3 PATTERN	3@$12	$36	XXX
CUFF LINKS	1 BASIC PAIR	$25	$25	
COLLAR	1 STRAIGHT BAR	$10	$10	
BAR	1 SAFETY-PIN	$10	$10	

TOTAL: $2,894

*New pieces must be added as budget allows

B | "Don'ts" for Men— Things to Work On

Tinted Glasses Indoors
They make you appear insincere; you don't need the handicap.

✖

Seven Hairs Across the Top
If you are losing your hair, admit it. Making those seven hairs work overtime isn't going to fool anyone.

✖

Short Sleeves at the Office
It just doesn't work. Period.

✖

Too Long Shirt Sleeves
Your sleeves should extend only 1/2 inch beyond your jacket.

✖

Jacket Too Small
If there are horizontal lines, the vent pulls open, or if the front button becomes a lethal weapon should you sneeze— it is just too small.

✖

Lapel Popping
When the lapels bow away from your chest, your jacket is either the wrong model or it is too small.

✖

Suspenders Worn with a Belt
Yikes! Unless you are tremendously insecure—never, never, never!

✖

High Water Pants
Forget the Johnstown Floods— pants must come down to cover your socks

✖

Fear of Pleats
Anyone can wear pleats if they are fitted properly. Give them a try, they are going to be around a long time.

✖

Lobster Bib Ties
The width of your tie should match the width of your lapel.

✖

Tie Too Short
Your tie should reach your belt line. This is neither arbitrary nor negotiable. Too short of a tie makes you look like a rube

Tie Clips and Tie Tacks
Dated. There are better ways to keep your tie out of your soup.

Ornate Belt Buckles
If it resembles an Inca sun god, you should not be wearing it to work.

Grandfather Clocks on Your Wrist
No bells, whistles or signal flares to mark the quarter hour.

Too Much Jewelry
The "Rule of Seven" applies to men as well as to women.

Cheap Briefcases
A briefcase says too much about you. Buy the best you can afford. It will serve you well for years.

Belted Trench Coats
Wear the belt knotted or stuffed into pockets. It looks too stiff to belt the coat "properly."

Black Socks with Everything
There is no rule that says you must wear black socks. Try gray socks with gray suits and navy with navy. Subtle patterns are hot, give them a try.

Exposing Your Shins
Please don't do this. Wear socks that are long enough.

Polishing Your Shoes with a Hershey Bar and a Brick
People make judgments about you based on your shoes. Take time to properly care for your shoes.

Alligators Nipping at Your Heels
If you can fit the eraser end of a pencil under your heel, it needs repair.

C | Finally— The Real Answers

1. See Chapter 11 for the hairstyle appropriate for your face shape.

2. Some of the hair replacement systems currently available today work for people who are prematurely losing their hair. A young head of hair on an old face does not look natural, so don't try to turn back the clock too far by using a toupee or "system."

3. No more than 20% tint is proper, preferably graduated.

4. If you cannot insert one finger between your neck and shirt, your collar it is too tight.

5. The skirt of a jacket should fully cover your seat.

6. Cuffs are recommended for dress trousers.

7. Trouser bottoms should reach the shoe tops.

8. Never wear a belt and braces (suspenders) together.

9. The width of your tie and lapel should be the same.

10. The wide end of the tie is always longer.

11. A small, conservative, gold toned buckle is always correct.

12. A leather briefcase regardless of style is best.

13. Socks should be long enough to cover the shins when seated with legs crossed. So mid or over the calf are best.

14. If you can slide the eraser end of a pencil under the heel they need to be replaced.

15. After the clippers it is the emery board.

16. The four-in-hand knot fits most shirt collar styles.

17. Identify, isolate, amplify and coordinate.

18. When worn with sportswear.

19. Puff, flop, TV fold and three point folds.

20. French cuffs are dressier.

✳ ✳ ✳

Knowledge is of two kinds:
we know a subject ourselves,
or we know where we can find
information upon it.

—Samuel Johnson
Boswell's *Life of Samuel Johnson*

D | How to Tie a Tie

THE FOUR-IN-HAND

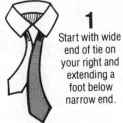

1 Start with wide end of tie on your right and extending a foot below narrow end.

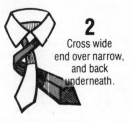

2 Cross wide end over narrow, and back underneath.

THE HALF WINDSOR

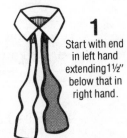

1 Start with wide end of tie on your right and extending a foot below narrow end.

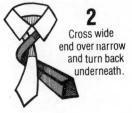

2 Cross wide end over narrow and turn back underneath.

THE BOW TIE

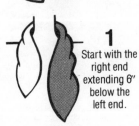

1 Start with end in left hand extending 1½" below that in right hand.

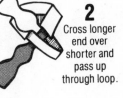

2 Cross longer end over shorter and pass up through loop.

THE ASCOT

1 Start with the right end extending 6" below the left end.

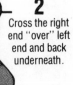

2 Cross the right end "over" left end and back underneath.

TIE TYING ILLUSTRATIONS

The ability to tie your necktie in more than one way is the mark of a truly skilled gentleman. These drawings are to be used as visual enhancements to the verbal instructions given earlier.

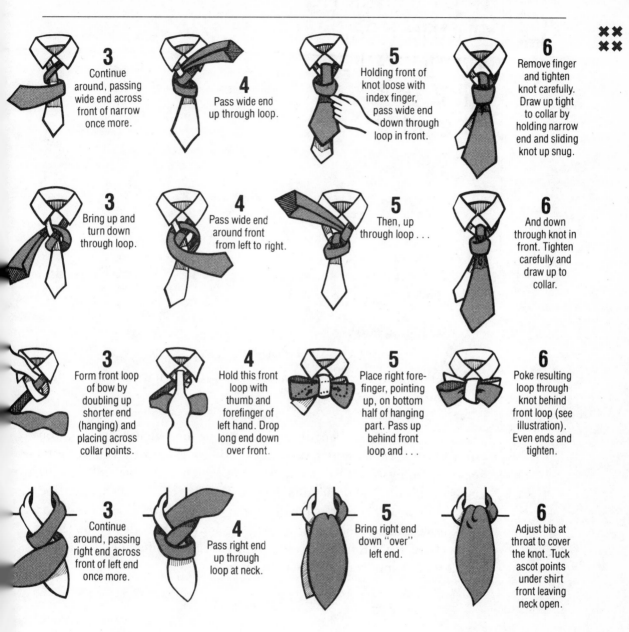

3 Continue around, passing wide end across front of narrow once more.

4 Pass wide end up through loop.

5 Holding front of knot loose with index finger, pass wide end down through loop in front.

6 Remove finger and tighten knot carefully. Draw up tight to collar by holding narrow end and sliding knot up snug.

3 Bring up and turn down through loop.

4 Pass wide end around front from left to right.

5 Then, up through loop . . .

6 And down through knot in front. Tighten carefully and draw up to collar.

3 Form front loop of bow by doubling up shorter end (hanging) and placing across collar points.

4 Hold this front loop with thumb and forefinger of left hand. Drop long end down over front.

5 Place right forefinger, pointing up, on bottom half of hanging part. Pass up behind front loop and . . .

6 Poke resulting loop through knot behind front loop (see illustration). Even ends and tighten.

3 Continue around, passing right end across front of left end once more.

4 Pass right end up through loop at neck.

5 Bring right end down "over" left end.

6 Adjust bib at throat to cover the knot. Tuck ascot points under shirt front leaving neck open.

Illustrations provided courtesy of Robert Talbott—The Talbott Studio, Carmel Valley, California.

E | Prior to Taking on the Real World: A Last Minute Checklist

Going out the door and taking a long, last look at yourself in a mirror has only three options as an outcome:

1. Everything is A–O.K.
2. Stop! Fix what you see before you leave.
3. OOPS! I never noticed that; I'll have to get that taken care of soon.

Examined in a full-length mirror and gone through item by item, you will never be unpleasantly surprised during an important meeting or appointment by what you or others see. In time the checklist will become an invaluable tool as you continually look for areas that need attention and then repair them as soon as possible. In a matter of weeks this pre-flight checklist will take no more than a few seconds to go through and soon after that will become automatic. In fact, you will begin running the checklist on people with whom you ride up in the elevator.

✖✖
✖✖

✖✖ **EXAMPLES OF #2—CAN AND SHOULD BE TAKEN CARE OF RIGHT AWAY**

Hair:

❏ Neatly combed and trimmed

Eyeglasses:

❏ Clean
❏ Not in need of repair

Nose and Ear Hair:

❏ Trimmed

Shirt:

❏ No cracked or missing bottoms
❏ Buttons easily (not too tight) at the neck
❏ Is fresh from the laundry and properly pressed
❏ No ink stains at pocket

Face:

❏ No shaving cuts with tissue attached
❏ Mustache/beard combed and neatly trimmed

Jacket:

❏ Buttons easily
❏ No loose threads
❏ Vent doesn't pull open
❏ Lapels lie flat on the chest

❏ No missing buttons
❏ No dandruff on the shoulders
❏ Neatly pressed

Trousers:

❏ Waist band fits comfortably
❏ Pant bottoms reach shoes tops
❏ Zipper fastened
❏ No belt if wearing suspenders
❏ Neatly pressed—no wrinkling at knees or lap
❏ Seat not shiny from excessive wear
❏ Cuffs and hem not frayed or hanging down

Tie:

❏ Reaches belt line
❏ Correct knot type for shirt collar
❏ No spots
❏ No creases
❏ No perspiration stains at the top of the knot

Belt:

❏ Fastened in middle holes
❏ Leather not worn where buckle has rubbed
❏ Coordinates with shoe color

Pocket Squares:

❑ Folded properly
❑ Blends with (not matches) the tie
❑ Pressed (not wrinkled from use)

Watch:

❑ Business not sport style

Briefcase:

❑ Dark or neutral belting leather
❑ Not seriously worn or scuffed

Trench/Overcoat:

❑ Falls below the knees
❑ Is wrinkle free

❑ Over the calf
❑ No holes
❑ Both same color
❑ Matches either trouser or shoe-color

Shoes:

❑ Highly polished
❑ No worn heels
❑ No holes in soles
❑ No patched lace
❑ Color matches/blends with suit/trouser color

✖✖ EXAMPLES OF #3: NEED PROFESSIONAL HELP OR REPLACEMENT—SOON

Wrinkles in the Coat:

❑ At the elbows
❑ On the top of the shoulder
❑ The suit skirt where it was sat on
❑ At the lapels if there's puckering

Trousers that Wrinkle and Sag:

❑ Bagging in the seat
❑ Wrinkling behind the knees
❑ Creases across the lap from sitting

Wrinkles in the Coat:

❑ At the elbows
❑ On the top of the shoulder
❑ The suit skirt where it was sat on
❑ At the lapels if there's puckering

Trousers that Wrinkle and Sag:

❑ Bagging in the seat
❑ Wrinkling behind the knees
❑ Creases across the lap from sitting

Shirt Collar Exposed:

❑ Too little collar above the jacket showing
❑ Too much collar showing (one-half to three-fourths inches is just right)

Jacket Collar Anchoring Correctly:

❑ No gap between the shirt and jacket collar

Trouser Bottoms-Length:

❑ Cuffs should break in front
❑ Plain bottoms slant back toward the heel

Shirt Cuff Showing:

❑ Not enough shirt sleeve (less than one-half inch)
❑ Too much shirt sleeve (three-fourths inch or more)

Correct Jacket Length:

❑ Reaches the curl of your fingers
❑ Covers your bottom
❑ Is half the distance from collar to floor

Index

Career
Resources

Contact Impact Publications to receive a free copy of their latest comprehensive and annotated catalog of career resources.

The following career resources are available directly from Impact Publications. Complete the following form or list the titles, include postage (see formula at the end), enclose payment, and send your order to:

IMPACT PUBLICATIONS
9104-N Manassas Drive
Manassas Park, VA 22111
Tel. 703/361-7300
FAX 703/335-9486

Orders from individuals must be prepaid by check, moneyorder, Visa or MasterCard number. We accept telephone and FAX orders with a Visa or MasterCard number.

Qty	TITLES	PRICE	TOTAL

DRESS, APPEARANCE, IMAGE

___	John Molloy's New Dress for Success	$10.95	___
___	Red Socks Don't Work	$14.95	___

JOB SEARCH STRATEGIES AND TACTICS

___	Change Your Job, Change Your Life	$14.95	___
___	Complete Job Finder's Guide to the 90s	$13.95	___
___	Dynamite Tele-Search	$10.95	___
___	Electronic Job Search Revolution	$12.95	___
___	Five Secrets to Finding a Job	$12.95	___
___	How to Get Interviews From Classified Job Ads	$14.95	___
___	Professional's Job Finder	$18.95	___

BEST JOBS AND EMPLOYERS FOR THE 90S

___	100 Best Companies to Work for in America	$27.95	___
___	American Almanac of Jobs and Salaries	$17.00	___
___	Best Jobs for the 1990s and Into the 21st Century	$12.95	___
___	Job Seeker's Guide to 1000 Top Employers	$22.95	___
___	Jobs Rated Almanac	$15.95	___
___	New Emerging Careers	$14.95	___

KEY DIRECTORIES

___	Career Training Sourcebook	$24.95	___
___	Dictionary of Occupational Titles	$39.95	___
___	Directory of Executive Recruiters (annual)	$44.95	___
___	Job Hunter's Sourcebook	$59.95	___
___	Moving and Relocation Directory	$149.00	___
___	National Directory of Addresses and Telephone Numbers	$129.95	___
___	National Trade and Professional Associations	$79.95	___
___	Occupational Outlook Handbook	$22.95	___
___	Places Rated Almanac	$21.95	___
___	Professional Careers Sourcebook	$79.95	___

CITY AND STATE JOB FINDERS (BOB ADAMS JOBBANKS)

___	Atlanta	$15.95	___
___	Boston	$15.95	___
___	Chicago	$15.95	___
___	Dallas/Fort Worth	$15.95	___
___	Denver	$15.95	___
___	Florida	$15.95	___
___	Houston	$15.95	___
___	Los Angeles	$15.95	___
___	Minneapolis	$15.95	___
___	New York	$15.95	___

___	Philadelphia	$15.95	_____
___	San Francisco	$15.95	_____
___	Seattle	$15.95	_____
___	Washington, DC	$15.95	_____

ALTERNATIVE JOBS AND CAREERS

___	Advertising Career Directory	$17.95	_____
___	Business and Finance Career Directory	$17.95	_____
___	But What If I Don't Want to Go to College?	$10.95	_____
___	Career Opportunities in the Sports Industry	$27.95	_____
___	Careers in Computers	$16.95	_____
___	Careers in Health Care	$16.95	_____
___	Environmental Career Guide	$14.95	_____
___	Marketing and Sales Career Directory	$17.95	_____
___	Outdoor Careers	$14.95	_____
___	Radio and Television Career Directory	$17.95	_____
___	Travel and Hospitality Career Directory	$17.95	_____

INTERNATIONAL, OVERSEAS, AND TRAVEL JOBS

___	Almanac of International Jobs and Careers	$14.95	_____
___	Complete Guide to International Jobs & Careers	$13.95	_____
___	Guide to Careers in World Affairs	$14.95	_____
___	How to Get a Job in Europe	$17.95	_____
___	Jobs for People Who Love Travel	$12.95	_____
___	Jobs in Russia and the Newly Independent States	$15.95	_____

PUBLIC-ORIENTED CAREERS

___	Almanac of American Government Jobs and Careers	$14.95	_____
___	Complete Guide to Public Employment	$19.95	_____
___	Federal Jobs in Law Enforcement	$15.95	_____
___	Find a Federal Job Fast!	$9.95	_____
___	Government Job Finder	$14.95	_____
___	Jobs and Careers With Nonprofit Organizations	$14.95	_____
___	The Right SF 171 Writer	$19.95	_____

JOB LISTINGS AND VACANCY ANNOUNCEMENTS

___	Federal Career Opportunities (6 biweekly issues)	$38.00	_____
___	International Employment Gazette (6 biweekly issues)	$35.00	_____
___	The Search Bulletin (6 issues)	$97.00	_____

SKILLS, TESTING, SELF-ASSESSMENT

___	Discover the Best Jobs for You	$11.95	_____
___	Do What You Love, the Money Will Follow	$10.95	_____
___	What Color Is Your Parachute?	$14.95	_____

Qty	TITLES	PRICE	TOTAL

RESUMES, LETTERS, AND NETWORKING

Qty	TITLES	PRICE	TOTAL
___	Dynamite Cover Letters	$9.95	_____
___	Dynamite Resumes	$9.95	_____
___	Electronic Resume Revolution	$12.95	_____
___	Electronic Resumes for the New Job Market	$11.95	_____
___	Great Connections	$11.95	_____
___	High Impact Resumes and Letters	$12.95	_____
___	Job Search Letters That Get Results	$12.95	_____
___	New Network Your Way to Job and Career Success	$12.95	_____

INTERVIEWS AND SALARY NEGOTIATIONS

Qty	TITLES	PRICE	TOTAL
___	60 Seconds and You're Hired!	$9.95	_____
___	Dynamite Answers to Interview Questions	$9.95	_____
___	Dynamite Salary Negotiation	$12.95	_____
___	Interview for Success	$11.95	_____
___	Sweaty Palms	$9.95	_____

MILITARY

Qty	TITLES	PRICE	TOTAL
___	From Army Green to Corporate Gray	$13.95	_____
___	Job Search: Marketing Your Military Experience	$14.95	_____
___	Re-Entry	$13.95	_____
___	Retiring From the Military	$22.95	_____

WOMEN AND SPOUSES

Qty	TITLES	PRICE	TOTAL
___	Doing It All Isn't Everything	$19.95	_____
___	New Relocating Spouse's Guide to Employment	$14.95	_____
___	Resumes for Re-Entry: A Handbook for Women	$10.95	_____
___	Survival Guide for Women	$16.95	_____

MINORITIES AND DISABLED

Qty	TITLES	PRICE	TOTAL
___	Best Companies for Minorities	$12.00	_____
___	Directory of Special Programs for Minority Group Members	$31.95	
___	Job Strategies for People With Disabilities	$14.95	_____
___	Minority Organizations	$49.95	_____
___	Work, Sister, Work	$19.95	_____

ENTREPRENEURSHIP AND SELF-EMPLOYMENT

Qty	TITLES	PRICE	TOTAL
___	101 Best Businesses to Start	$15.00	_____
___	Best Home-Based Businesses for the 90s	$10.95	_____
___	Entrepreneur's Guide to Starting a Successful Business	$16.95	_____
___	Have You Got What It Takes?	$12.95	_____

ORDER FORM SUBTOTAL　　　　　　　　　　　　　　_____

Virginia residents add 4% sales tax　　　　　　　_____

POSTAGE/HANDLING ($3.00 for first
title and $1.00 for each additional book)　　　_$3.00_　　✸✸ ✸✸

Number of additional titles x $1.00　　　　　　_____

TOTAL ENCLOSED　　　　　　　　　　　　　_____

NAME_____

ADDRESS_____

_____

_____

❑ I enclose check/moneyorder for $_____ made payable

to IMPACT PUBLICATIONS.

❑ Please charge $_____ to my credit card:

Card #_____

Expiration date _____ /_____

Signature _____

■ ▬ ■ ▬ ■ ▬ ■ ▬ ■ ▬ ■ ▬ ■ ▬ ■ ▬ ■ ▬ ■ ▬ ■ ▬ ■ ▬

SEMINARS AND WORKSHOPS

For more information about the author's Personal Packaging presentation
for the men and women of your organization, please send your name,
address, and phone and fax numbers to

KENCAY INTERNATIONAL
1800 Old Meadow Rd. #502
McLean, VA 22102

NAME _____

ADDRESS _____

CITY _____ STATE _____ ZIP _____

TEL_____ FAX _____